Silent Cells

Also by Anthony Ryan Hatch
Published by the University of Minnesota Press

Blood Sugar: Racial Pharmacology and Food Justice in Black America

SILENT CELLS

The Secret Drugging of Captive America

ANTHONY RYAN HATCH

University of Minnesota Press
Minneapolis
London

The publication of this book was assisted by a bequest from Josiah H. Chase to honor his parents, Ellen Rankin Chase and Josiah Hook Chase, Minnesota territorial pioneers.

The University of Minnesota Press gratefully acknowledges financial assistance for the publication of this book from the Dean of the Social Sciences and the Center for African American Studies at Wesleyan University.

Portions of the Introduction were previously published as Anthony Ryan Hatch and Kym Bradley, "Prisons Matter: Psychotropics and the Trope of Silence in Technocorrections," in *Mattering: Feminism, Science, and Materialism,* ed. Victoria Pitts-Taylor (New York: New York University Press, 2016), 224–44. Portions of chapter 4 were previously published as Anthony Ryan Hatch, Marik Xavier-Brier, Brandon Atell, and Eryn Viscarra, "Soldier, Elder, Prisoner, Ward: Psychotropics in the Era of Transinstitutionalization," in *Advances in Medical Sociology, Volume 17. Fifty Years after Deinstitutionalization: Mental Illness in Contemporary Communities,* ed. Brea L. Perry (Bingley, U.K.: Emerald Publishing Group), 291–317; reprinted with permission of Emerald Publishing Group.

Published by the University of Minnesota Press
111 Third Avenue South, Suite 290
Minneapolis, MN 55401–2520
http://www.upress.umn.edu

Printed in the United States of America on acid-free paper

The University of Minnesota is an equal-opportunity educator and employer.

25 24 23 22 21 20 19   10 9 8 7 6 5 4 3 2 1

Library of Congress Cataloging-in-Publication Data
Names: Hatch, Anthony Ryan, author.
Title: Silent cells : the secret drugging of captive America / Anthony Ryan Hatch.
Description: Minneapolis : University of Minnesota Press, [2019] | Includes
   bibliographical references and index. |
Identifiers: LCCN 2018045727 (print) | ISBN 978-1-5179-0743-3 (hc) |
   ISBN 978-1-5179-0744-0 (pb)
Subjects: LCSH: Prisoners—Health and hygiene—United States. | Mentally ill
   prisoners—United States. | Psychotropic drugs—United States. | Mental illness—
   Treatment—Moral and ethical aspects—United States. | Corrections—United States.
Classification: LCC HV8843 .H38 2019 (print) | DDC 365/.66720973—dc23
LC record available at https://lccn.loc.gov/2018045727

*This book is dedicated to the millions of people the world over
who experience bondage of mind and body
and to those millions more who yearn
for their immediate, unconditional, and permanent liberation*

CONTENTS

I began the investigations that would turn into this book during a 2009 National Institute of Mental Health (NIMH) fellowship at the Morehouse School of Medicine in Atlanta. The fellowship was focused on mental health, substance use, and HIV/AIDS in correctional settings, and experts in the field of correctional health made scholarly presentations that were supposed to help the fellows get the lay of the land in prison health research. Occasionally, the conversations took interesting turns. One day, a former prison psychiatrist came to visit. She was a well-dressed African American woman who had recently left the Georgia Department of Corrections for work in greener pastures as an executive at a for-profit prison health care corporation. After her talk, I asked her what she thought about the use of psychotropic drugs inside America's prisons. *Psychotropics* is an umbrella term for prescription drugs that change brain chemistry and affect the functioning of the central nervous system; such drugs are prescribed routinely across the United States to treat everything from everyday emotional problems to serious psychiatric disorders. They include the antidepressants, antipsychotics, mood stabilizers, stimulants, and tranquilizers that an alarming number of citizens, both free and unfree, take on a daily basis. The former prison psychiatrist, now prison profiteer, rocked back on her heels, gave a wry smirk, and replied, "Each year, the warden would send me and my staff a nice bottle of something, because he knew we kept the prison quiet."

Her candor was striking, sparking my curiosity about the role that psychotropic drugs might play not just in maintaining mass incarceration but also in generating new modes of neurobiological control over people's minds—and lives. Psychotropics keep prisons quiet? The good doctor's response suggested that mental health staff, working in close consultation with guards and administrators, administer psychotropic drugs to prisoners not only to treat their mental illnesses but also to ensure that they are more docile, more compliant, less likely to cause trouble or be violent. Is that really how the system works? Or was she just being hyperbolic in an insider conversation among experts in training? Even the suggestion that prisons might use psychotropics for the purpose of silencing prisoners, both sociologically and mentally, reflected a sinister injustice that I was not prepared to accept. That moment was the genesis for this book.

I wanted to know how prisons use psychotropics—in particular, I wanted to know if there was any truth to what the former prison psychiatrist had said. In pursuing the question, however, I found that I faced a number of barriers. First, it was made clear that the main objective of the NIMH fellowship was for the fellows to design science projects that the National Institutes of Health would consider worthy of funding and that would lead to a series of liberal reforms designed to improve various features of American prison systems' approaches to health. The other fellows and I were all early-career professors of color (we were all African American), and we were encouraged to develop politically safe projects that would lead to federal funding, peer-reviewed research articles, tenure, and other professional rewards. All of that sounded sweet, especially to new young research professors who wanted economic and professional security, but I had an uncomfortable feeling that our science was supposed to be intended to benefit us first. Then, if we were both smart and lucky, our work might, at some point in the future, lead to better institutional policies in prisons and improved health outcomes for prisoners. In other words, we were encouraged to create liberal science that could be used to achieve liberal health policy reform. For example, we might design an intervention to encourage prisoners to make better health choices. Or we might study postrelease planning services that help formerly incarcerated people reenter society. Many of the fellows pursued solid liberal projects like these—and there is definitely a place in the world for good liberal science.

But I did not want to participate in liberal science. I wanted to do *liberatory* social science that would challenge whatever made the uniquely American version of mass imprisonment possible. Earlier that year, I had completed a dissertation that formed the basis for my book *Blood Sugar: Racial Pharmacology and Food Justice in Black America,* and I recognized through that work that I was not at all interested in doing liberal social science.[1] My aim in that project was not to improve the science of metabolic syndrome; rather, I wanted to end the science of metabolic syndrome, or at least end its racist variations. Similarly, it seemed an unconscionable waste of time to design a science project focused on prison health that would only tinker with certain aspects of the prison health care system. All of the fellows knew that U.S. prisons were part of a vast and violent system of social and political control; the practices of the associated network of private prison health care companies and vendors just compounded the injustices of the system. I could not bear the thought of producing scholarship that aimed merely to reform this system.

Strangely, few feminist and critical race scholars who study science and technology have examined the prison as a site of the enmeshing of natures and cultures made possible through technoscience. By allowing the technoscientific practices that support mass incarceration to remain unquestioned, the field of science and technology studies remains politically disengaged from one of the most important struggles for human freedom in our time. This oversight is curious given the centrality of philosopher Michel Foucault's work to political analyses of technoscience. Foucault theorized the prison as a "complete" or "austere" institution that manufactures disciplined bodies through a tightly coordinated system of architectural structures, social practices, and institutional procedures.[2]

The second barrier that I faced, linked to this question of liberal science, was methodological. I imagined the futility and frustration of seeking admission to prisons to interview officials and mental health providers about any punitive, unethical, nonmedical drugging of prisoners. What prison officials in their right minds would ever admit to unethical or unconstitutional psychotropic drugging practices? Beyond that impossibility, the methodological challenge of studying practices inside prisons opened up a new line of inquiry for me. I began to envision a study that would try to document what we know and do not know about the use of psychotropics in prisons and would consider only publicly available sources as evidence. Imprisonment is carried out in the name of protecting the citizenry and is done with the public's consent. The government pays the bills for prisons, and we, as citizens, sign the checks that pay for prisoners' medical care, including psychotropics, and the entirety of the system. What information had the government provided its citizens about psychotropic drugs in prisons? What had other scientists and activists and advocates uncovered?

I began to wonder what a reasonably well-trained scientist-citizen could uncover about the use of psychotropics in U.S. prisons without speaking to any prison officials or health care providers directly. While I knew that there were good people with good hearts working ethically within prisons, I was not interested in their opinions and beliefs about prisoners' psychotropic drug use. I wanted to evaluate what the documentary record said and did not say about the practice. I searched the biomedical and social science research literature, usually an archive full of information, but I didn't have much luck. I traveled to the National Library of Medicine, housed at the National Institutes of Health in Bethesda, Maryland, and found surprisingly little there about psychotropics in prisons. Even the Bureau of Justice Statistics, the government agency responsible for producing and compiling data on criminal justice in the United States, had produced only a few official reports, based on limited prison surveys, on the subject of psychotropics, and these left many questions unanswered. Even some very basic questions could not be answered because there were no sources of data that could be analyzed to answer them.

For instance, when did prisons start giving psychotropic drugs to prisoners, and why? How were the drugs administered exactly, and how did prisons control the flow of their pharmaceutical inventories? Which drugs were distributed in prisons, and why those drugs and not others? Which prisoners were given drugs, and why? What role did psychiatry and diagnoses of mental illness play in this process? And, most important for me, what evidence existed to indicate that psychotropics were being used to silence people living in state custody?

To my great shock, these questions had not been addressed anywhere in a systematic way. As I looked for other scholars' answers to these questions and considered a wide range of source material for this project, I began to encounter troubling linkages between the ways in which prisons might be using psychotropic drugs to silence populations of prisoners and the use of psychotropics in other sectors of the "carceral state"—nursing homes, the foster care system, the active-duty military, immigrant detention facilities, the schools that educate our children. I knew that psychotropics had become ubiquitous in American society, but was I onto something much bigger? Had these drugs become a mode of control and pacification not limited to prisoners but affecting the entirety of captive America? This book represents my effort to figure that out.

Psychotropics may serve to keep the prisons quiet, but if we listen carefully, we can also hear the clarion call for transformation of America's prison system. In a movement harking back to the prison abolition movements of the 1960s and 1970s, millions of Americans, led by organizations like Critical Resistance, are now calling for an end to mass incarceration in the United States. In his last year in office, President Obama commuted the sentences of many nonviolent drug offenders, and both of his attorneys general, Eric Holder and Loretta Lynch, seemed to be on the side of solid liberal sentencing reform. In 2014, the U.S. Sentencing Commission added its weighty opinion to arguments for changes in the mandatory sentencing guidelines for nonviolent drug offenses, which have, in large part, been responsible for the ballooning of federal prison populations over the past forty years.[3] Even in the era of Donald Trump, bipartisan coalitions have called for reforms that may serve to slow the rate of incarceration, reduce prison terms, and begin to rethink the U.S. prison system. We can hear the voices calling for change. Will our political leaders listen? Will they, for once, have the courage to act in the name of freedom?

INTRODUCTION

INCARCERATING BODIES AND BRAINS

If you've ever been to a prison or jail—and if you're poor and brown in America the chances are better than they should be that you have—you know that they are loud places. Doors slam, people yell, guards bark, and bells ring. The absence of sound-absorbent building materials, like carpet and drywall, means that sounds echo against structures of concrete, steel, and riot-proof Plexiglas. The constant noise makes doing hard time even harder.

It may seem to many readers that the story of mass incarceration in the United States has already been told—this nation has the highest incarceration rate in the world and imprisons poor people, especially black and Latino men, disproportionately. More than 2 million people are held in prisons and jails across the United States, and millions more are on probation or parole. Currently some 400,000 foreign nationals are being held in privately run immigrant detention facilities, and 2.3 million other immigrants must check in with the government on a routine basis, many of them unsure if they will be deported. More than 10,000 immigrant children are being detained in massive tent cities. Hundreds if not thousands more individuals are incarcerated in war-zone prisons maintained by the U.S. military and other national security institutions. But what if we extend our conception of what it means to be confined to a much broader set of institutions that includes any that people are not exactly able to leave physically of their own volition? The state confines citizens in many places other than prisons. Take, for example, the roughly 400,000 young people who are in the custody of the foster care system.[1] Or the millions of people serving in the armed forces, who cannot exactly go AWOL. What about the millions of elders living in government-regulated and -subsidized nursing homes? In American society today, a great many people exist, if not in actual prison cells, in spaces they are not exactly free to leave.

Let's call this broader system of confinement *captive America*; it consists of a vast and interconnected network of total institutions that are subject to federal, state, and local governance. Sociologist Erving Goffman famously used Everett Hughes's concept of the total institution to describe these highly rational and bureaucratic institutions, which are closed off in various ways from so-called free society.[2] Total institutions have three principal organizational features: all aspects of life within them are highly regulated under one official authority, inmates are required to do the same activities together in public, and "the various enforced activities are brought together into a single rational plan purportedly designed to fulfill the official aims of the institution."[3] According to Goffman, there are five types of total institutions: (1) welfare institutions for the blind, the aged, the orphaned, and the indigent; (2) medical institutions for persons in need of inpatient physical or mental health care (e.g., tuberculosis sanitariums and mental hospitals); (3) penal institutions such as prisons, jails, concentration camps, and war camps; (4) institutions organized around specific kinds of work and labor (e.g., army barracks, ships, boarding schools, work campuses, colonial compounds, large mansions); and (5) religious training and practice institutions (e.g., abbeys, monasteries, convents, and cloisters).[4] These institutions diminish the identities of the individuals within them, restructure their social roles and identities, and make them unfit for the outside world through a series of rituals enacted through admission, treatment, and social interactions with staff.[5] Through these transformations, total institutions are "the forcing houses for changing persons," each one a "natural experiment on what can be done to the self."[6]

Goffman believed that total institutions serve as "storage dumps" for society's outcasts.[7] The great contradiction of total institutions lies in the tension between their professed goals (e.g., caring for the mentally or physically ill, protecting the aged or vulnerable, guarding the dangerous) and their undeclared use as dumping grounds.[8] As they conform to changing cultural ideas about what constitutes care, total institutions work on people in ways that tend to conflict with the need for the bureaucratic efficiencies and controlled costs associated with warehousing large numbers of people. In other words, the hypocrisy between what total institutions say they do to people and what they actually do is measured in changes in people's bodies and in the institutions' accounting for money spent or saved. In order for people to be warehoused in these storage dumps, they must be transformed into things that can be stored at a reasonable price.

What if the new plan for governing and controlling the millions of people forced to live in captive America is to move them from their institutional cells to new locations *inside their own brain cells,* into mental prisons that perform the same work as the old physical prisons or barracks or hospital rooms, but with new technologies of pacification? This would be a new kind of prison cell indeed. This is where an untold story about how we achieve mass incarceration begins.

Psychotropic drugs are widely distributed in so-called free society to help people cope with what are commonly understood to be mental or psychiatric illnesses. Reducing (and ultimately eliminating) racial and gender inequalities in access to mental health care has become a central priority of U.S. health care institutions, policies, and researchers. Enabling equitable access to mental health treatment has proven to be an especially pernicious problem given the individual, cultural, and economic factors that structure access to health care in general in the United States. Indeed, members of racial and ethnic minority groups are less likely than whites to report receiving any mental health treatment, counseling, or medication.[9] Paradoxically, racial and ethnic minorities report lower rates of mental illness. Both of these findings may be attributed at least in part to differences in socioeconomic status. That is, lower-income minorities may have limited access to the health insurance and financial resources necessary to offset the cost of mental health care, and higher-income whites may be more aggressive in obtaining mental health care and treatment.

As noted in the Preface, psychotropics encompass several subclasses of prescription drugs (antipsychotics, antidepressants, mood stabilizers, stimulants, and antianxiety drugs) that change brain chemistry and affect the functioning of the brain and the central nervous system. In recent decades, psychotropic drug use has increased steadily among noninstitutionalized adolescents and adults.[10] It is surprisingly hard to get recent data on this question, but researchers who analyzed a nationally representative sample of adults from the 2013 Medical Expenditure Panel Survey estimated that 16.7 percent of adult Americans were taking at least one psychotropic drug—about one out of six people.[11] White people have been found to be twice as likely as people of color, and women twice as likely as men, to take psychotropics, and 80 percent of users report long-term use. General practitioners, who are not typically trained to recognize and diagnose mental illnesses, are more likely than psychiatrists to prescribe psychotropics to patients and to keep patients on psychotropics longer.[12] Yet, even when they are prescribed and used in ways consistent with gold-standard psychiatric practice, psychotropic drugs are associated with suicide, homicide, and other forms of interpersonal violence.[13]

Critics have questioned the effectiveness, overall safety, and clinical appropriateness of psychotropics for treating mental health problems in noninstitutional settings.[14] Exactly how psychotropics affect the brain, how they actually transform the human body, is not known, but clearly they do "work" by interacting with brain and body. Scholars in the field of social studies of science, technology, and medicine frame pharmaceuticals as biotechnologies that actively mediate the relationship between human bodies and cultural systems, particularly along the axes of gender and race.[15] The positioning of psychotropics as biotechnologies opens up the investigation of these drugs beyond questions about the intentions of patients as they consume direct-to-consumer advertising or health care professionals as they prescribe drugs under pressure from pharmaceutical companies. I take the view that psychotropics are not merely "tools" that social actors use to achieve particular effects; they are technologies that have agency in the world in large measure through the ways in which they transform the brains and bodies of those who ingest them.

In this book, I argue that psychotropics have become central not only to mass incarceration in prisons but also to other kinds of mass captivity within the U.S. carceral state. I address one big counterfactual question: *Is it possible for the U.S. carceral state to exist without psychotropics?* Answering this question requires thinking about the material effects that psychotropic drugs have on human brains and bodies and interrogating the systematic production of knowledge about how psychotropics are used in captive America. My central argument is that psychotropic drugs manufacture two kinds of silent cells: one at the level of the bodies and brains of captive people and the other at the level of knowledge about the material effects of those drugs on people. These two interlocking meanings of *silent cells* permeate this book.

PSYCHOTROPICS AND THE RISE OF THE CARCERAL STATE

Alongside the explosion in prescription psychotropic use, since the 1980s, the United States has experienced unparalleled growth in prison structures, populations, and industries. At the end of 1980, there were 319,598 persons incarcerated in state and federal prisons.[16] By 2014, the number had swelled to an alarming 1,574,700.[17] Including those in jails and on probation, currently more than 2.3 million people are under penal control in the United States, which now incarcerates a greater percentage of its citizens than any other nation in recorded history. The exponential growth in prison construction and prison-related industries has created an entirely new sector of the U.S. economy.[18] Further, the ubiquity of prisons in U.S. popular culture—in movies, television, and popular music—has contributed to the seeming permanence of mass incarceration.[19] Simultaneously, prisons have become "the new asylums," warehousing hundreds of thousands of men and women who experience mental illness; for some, mental illness preceded their detention, but for many others, it emerged as a result of their imprisonment.[20] It is estimated that well over half of all people incarcerated in federal, state, and jail facilities in the United States suffer from some form of psychic distress. Today, there are more people with serious psychiatric illness in prisons than there are in America's remaining psychiatric hospitals.[21]

At the turn of the millennium, the administration of psychotropic drugs was the most prevalent and often the only form of mental health practice available in U.S. prisons.[22] Currently, doctors routinely prescribe psychotropics to prisoners for a wide range of reasons, some of which are related to the treatment of psychosocial symptoms and psychiatric disorders and some of which are linked to the need to maintain order. According to a federal census of state prisons in 2000, 73 percent of state prisons were distributing psychotropic drugs to their prisoners— this was the most common form of mental health treatment, followed by initial mental health screening (70 percent), therapy/counseling (71 percent), referrals to mental health services upon reentry (66 percent), psychiatric assessments (65 percent), and twenty-four-hour mental health care (51 percent). The institutional use of psychotropics has been found to be positively related to increasing levels of confinement: in 2000, 95 percent of maximum/high-security state prisons distributed psychotropics, compared to 88 percent of medium-security prisons and 62 percent of minimum/low-security prisons.[23]

Data from the 2004 Survey of Inmates in State and Federal Correctional Facilities show that among inmates with previously diagnosed mental conditions who had been treated with psychotropic drugs before their incarceration, 69.1 percent of federal and 68.8 percent of state inmates received psychotropics during their incarceration.[24] In 2006, 46 percent of prisoners in Vermont's Department of Corrections were taking at least one psychotropic drug.[25] In 2009, more than 16,000 federal prisoners received psychotropics—7 percent of the total federal prison population.[26] In 2009, the Corrections Center of Northeast Ohio spent half of its medical budget on psychotropics.[27] In July 2002, Clark County Jail in Springfield, Ohio, spent more on psychotropics than it did on food.[28]

Psychotropics are a major element of the policy approach called *technocorrections,* the strategic application of new technologies in the effort to reduce the costs of mass incarceration and minimize the risks that prisoners pose to society.[29] Psychotropics, electronic tracking and location systems, and genetic and neurobiological risk assessments are all tools of technocorrections. Dr. Tony Fabelo, a prison policy strategist who now works for the Council of State Governments, coined the term in 2000. Here, he outlines the great potential of psychotropics as a tool of technocorrections:

> Pharmacological breakthroughs—new "wonder" drugs being developed to control behavior in correctional and noncorrectional settings—will also affect technocorrections. Correctional officials are already familiar with some of these drugs, as many are currently used to treat mentally ill offenders. *Yet these drugs could be easily used to control mental conditions affecting behaviors considered undesirable even when the offenders are not mentally ill. . . .*
>
> . . . These drugs could become correctional tools to manage violent offenders and perhaps even to prevent violence.[30]

Psychotropics are used not only to manage mental illness but also to help people cope with exposure to stressful institutional environments, like prisons.[31] We should expect prison health care policies to be organized with security and confinement in mind, even as these policies are also designed to provide minimum standards of care for the sick. In other words, even when a prisoner has serious mental health problems, the use of psychotropics always falls under the logic of control and submission that permeates the prison–prisoner relationship.[32] Yet technocorrections is not new.

We know little about the use of psychotropics in U.S. prisons prior to the penal reform movement of the 1970s that emerged in the wake of the 1971 riot at Attica Prison. In the 1970s, the use of tranquilizers in state mental hospitals and prisons became visible through journalists' investigations and high-profile legal cases.[33] Several legal analysts also drew attention to the problematic use of psychotropics in prisons, a topic that has received only scant coverage in the years since.[34] Prison officials are quick to point to a small number of cases that have been documented of prisoners abusing prescribed psychotropic medications, primarily the antipsychotic drug quetiapine (sold under the brand name Seroquel).[35] Back in 1974, Ted Morgan of the *New York Times* visited a notorious New York City detention facility known as the Tombs (because it was said to resemble an Egyptian tomb). As Morgan described it, the main function of the psychiatrist in the Tombs was to "drug the inmate into submissiveness and prevent suicide attempts." To the detainees who were awaiting trial, "the psychiatrist has become the successor of the brutal guard. Both men work toward the same goal: to produce a model prisoner, quiet and passive, who answers when he is spoken to and does what he is told. Where the brutal guard used rubber hoses, the psychiatrist relies on powerful tranquilizers like Thorazine." This double function of psychotropics is also mirrored in Morgan's observations about the cavalier practice of drugging: "A sure way to quiet down a man who is 'acting out' is to put him on 1,100 milligrams of Thorazine a day. It turns him into a zombie. Or, in clinical terms, it screens off the amount of input so the inmate can reorganize his psychic structure."[36] In 1980, a group of prisoners held in the U.S. penitentiary in Leavenworth, Kansas, wrote to Congress to protest unjust treatment by prison officials. They stated:

> The Leavenworth prison authorities utilize widespread forced drugging for completely inappropriate reasons; it could be fairly viewed as a preventive detention measure utilizing chemical strait jackets. . . .
> Some of us have tried to physically resist the injections—believing it inherently unjust to be given dangerous medication for certified psychotics when we're not psychotic—only to be assaulted by their "goon squad," beaten, held down, injected with Prolixin and confined in the neuropsychiatric ward. Some are resigned to our fate and regard it as futile to resist this *mad technototalitarianism*. We merely acquiesce to their demands and take our periodic injections quietly.[37]

In mobilizing a policy of technocorrections, prisons press human beings through the mold of prison culture, reifying relations of institutionalized racism and sexism.[38] The prison–industrial complex relies on and creates such relationships of power. The fact that American prisons are unjustly stratified by intersectional dynamics is beyond question.[39] By *intersectional dynamics,* I mean the ways in which social structures of race, gender, and class operate simultaneously to shape people's experiences, entire communities, and major social institutions.[40] Scholars have carefully analyzed how the institutional practices and cultural meanings that structure prison life are shaped by intersectional dynamics that operate through race, gender, social class, sexuality, nationality, and disability.[41] An intersectional approach provides an important framework for analysis because it rejects either/or thinking and embraces both/and thinking about the nature of relationships of power and resistance; this orientation asks us to interrogate the ways in which racism, sexism, and class inequality work together as complementary rather than competing explanations for mass captivity. As Angela Davis and Michelle Alexander have strenuously argued, the prison–industrial complex and the criminal injustice system that feeds it both rely on and inform these systems of power as they affect prisoners, their families and communities, and the entire nation.[42]

If psychotropics function as "chemical straitjackets," as the Leavenworth prisoners claimed, these drugs' production and consumption are shaped by gendered and racial meanings.[43] Prison psychiatrists are much more likely to prescribe psychotropics to female prisoners than to males, a fact related to higher rates of psychiatric diagnoses and symptomology among incarcerated women.[44] The presumed criminality of women in prison is also understood within the context of gender ideology organized around femininity and through the female body.[45] In 1976, a group of women imprisoned at the Bedford Hills Correctional Facility were strip-searched, shackled, and then transferred to the Matteawan State Hospital for the Criminally Insane in New York because they represented "disciplinary problems" for the prison. There, the women were drugged with antidepressants, antipsychotics, sedatives, and tranquilizers.[46] None of the women were ever diagnosed with any mental disorders, and they subsequently filed and won a civil case against the prison and the hospital, settling out of court for $4,857.14 each.[47] At the civil trial, hospital officials openly admitted that "medication often serves a dual purpose in the physical and mental rehabilitation of patients and inmates . . . toward both effective custody and effective rehabilitation."[48]

State-level research conducted by Renée Baillargeon and colleagues within the Texas prison system in the late 1990s showed that, in comparison with white prisoners, African American and Hispanic prisoners were more likely to receive older, more outdated antipsychotics and antidepressants or no pharmacotherapy at all.[49] In 1988, officials at Stateville Prison and Menard Hospital in Illinois forced Albert Sullivan, a black prisoner, to take large doses of haloperidol (Haldol), an antipsychotic drug. In subsequent legal proceedings, Sullivan alleged that Dr. Parwatikar, a psychiatrist, and Mary Flannigan, the superintendent at Menard, forced him to take powerful drugs "because of [his] black race, male sex, poverty and because I am a prisoner and mental patient and sex-offender." At trial, Dr. Parwatikar stated:

> The need for Mr. Sullivan being on anti-psychotic medication is quite clear from the past history. During the period of 1972 thru 1982 [he] had 59 assaultive episodes. Thus, it is quite essential that Mr. Sullivan must be on some sort of anti-psychotic medication for the rest of his life.[50]

Given the legal rules governing forced medication in Illinois, Sullivan was not able to stop taking the medication long enough to prove that he did not need it. As this case illustrates, the government's power to force psychotropic medication, people's rights of refusal, and the dynamics of psychiatric care are sometimes sorted out by the judicial system.

U.S. LAW AND THE USE OF PSYCHOTROPICS

In this book I also explore the complex relationships among state power, human rights, and citizenship that accompany the use of psychotropics in captive America. Prisoners occupy a unique position within U.S. law and psychiatric practice. Not fully citizens with all of the rights and entitlements guaranteed thereto, they exist in a precarious social location at the bottom of the U.S. civic structure. In fact, the status of prisoners challenges our commonsense understanding of citizenship in the United States. While convicted felons lose their freedom, the right to vote, the right to work in certain occupations, and the right to public benefits such as housing, they also gain new rights to health care, including mental health treatment. By receiving health care, prisoners exercise their constitutional right not to die as the result of deliberate indifference in prison. These new rights bring with them significant costs, however. By exercising the right to receive health care, prisoners open themselves up to poor-quality care, ethical abuses, medical negligence, and forced treatments. Psychotropics serve as a kind of boundary object through which we can evaluate the substantive meanings of what anthropologist Adriana Petryna calls biological citizenship.[51]

A number of laws and legal rulings provide some structure regarding the government's authority to distribute psychotropics to confined people. The U.S. Supreme Court's ruling in *Estelle v. Gamble* (1976) effectively established prisoners' right to access health care, their right to receive care ordered for them by officials, and their right to seek professional medical judgment.[52] Prisoners' right of access to health care includes the constitutional obligation of the prison to provide a minimum standard of mental health care to inmates. Perhaps surprisingly, prisoners are the only group in the United States who have a federal constitutional right to health care; soldiers and veterans are also guaranteed access to health care, but that guarantee is not covered by the U.S. constitution.

Although federal regulations and state laws do not explicitly enshrine a right to health care for so-called free persons, they do shape psychotropic drug use in the broader U.S. carceral state. For example, the *Code of Federal Regulations* protects the right of nursing home residents "to be free from any physical or chemical restraints imposed for purposes of discipline or convenience, and not required to treat the resident's medical symptoms."[53] State laws protect the right of children in foster care to receive adequate health care, including, as in the state of Texas, the right "not to be forced to take unnecessary or too much medication."[54]

One way in which the state asserts its custodial power over prisoners is by forcing them to take psychotropics, which it can do if a prisoner is classified as dangerous and if the forced drugging is deemed to be in the "best medical interest of the prisoner."[55] In the case of *Washington v. Harper* (1990), the U.S. Supreme Court examined two questions: Can the state administer antipsychotic drugs to prisoners involuntarily? And are there sufficient protections for prisoners in the policies that make such administration possible?[56] The court ruled that the government can administer psychotropics involuntarily to an inmate if it is determined that "he is a danger to himself or others and the treatment is in his medical interest." The court further found the Washington state policy under which inmate Walter Harper was forcibly medicated to be rational because "it applies exclusively to mentally ill inmates who are gravely disabled or represent a significant danger to themselves or others; the drugs may be administered only for treatment and under the direction of a licensed psychiatrist; and there is little dispute in the psychiatric profession that the proper use of the drugs is an effective means of treating and controlling a mental illness likely to cause violent behavior."[57] Prisoners can request review of the prison's decision to forcibly drug them, but such reviews are essentially in-house, conducted by prison medical officials, and tend to favor the decisions of prison officials.

Legal analysts interpret *Washington v. Harper* as a case involving "biological alteration," a process through which the "government transforms individuals into instruments of state policy."[58] Other biological alteration cases include *Buck v. Bell* (1927), which involved forced sterilization, and *Jacobson v. Massachusetts* (1905), which dealt with compulsory vaccination. These cases center on two key questions: What constitutes a biological alteration? And to what ends are the interventions deployed? In other words, what exactly is the government doing, and why is it doing it?

Prisoners can refuse to take psychotropics under certain legal conditions that affirm their constitutional rights to free speech, bodily integrity, and due process.[59] In *Riggins v. Nevada* (1992), the Supreme Court found that involuntary administration of psychotropics to a defendant violated that defendant's due process rights, but it could still be done.[60] In *Sell v. United States* (2003), the court affirmed the government's power to administer psychotropics to mentally ill defendants to make them competent to stand trial for serious criminal charges "if the treatment is medically appropriate, is substantially unlikely to have side effects that may undermine the trial's fairness, and, taking account of less intrusive alternatives, is necessary significantly to further important governmental trial-related interests."[61] Similarly, the court found in an earlier case that in certain circumstances the state can condition parole on the involuntary use of antipsychotic drugs, subject to appropriate procedural protections.[62] And, perhaps most alarmingly, government authorities have worked out ways to forcibly administer psychotropics to defendants to make them competent to stand trial when they are facing the death penalty.[63]

The case of *Nelson v. Heyne* (1974) involved several inmates of the Indiana Boys School who had brought a class action lawsuit against the institution for using the antipsychotics Sparine and Thorazine solely for the purpose of controlling inmates' excited behavior.[64] Boys weighing less than 116 pounds were given 25 milligrams of Sparine, and boys over that weight were given 50 milligrams of Sparine. The boys had not been examined by medically competent staff members and were not a part of a structured psychotherapeutic program. In its ruling, the Seventh Circuit Court of Appeals wrote:

> Major tranquilizing drugs are occasionally administered by the Defendants for the purpose of controlling excited behavior rather than as part of an ongoing, psycho-therapeutic program. Standing orders by the doctor at the Boys School permits the registered nurse and licensed practical nurse on duty to prescribe dosages of specified tranquilizers upon the recommendation of the custodial staff at the Boys School. The drugs are administered inter-muscularly. The facts show that there is no procedure utilized whereby medically competent staff members evaluate individuals to whom the drugs are administered, either before or after injections.[65]

The court found that the indiscriminate use of tranquilizers in this case violated the boys' Eighth Amendment protection against cruel and unusual punishment and their Fourteenth Amendment right to due process, noting that "the [Indiana Boys School] policies are far afield of minimal medical and constitutional standards."[66]

These legal cases demonstrate the meaninglessness of the boundary between psychiatric therapy and custodial control in prisons. During the 1970s, scholars investigated, and scholarly journals published articles about, isolated cases of the misuse of psychotropics, what Edward Opton, now a lawyer at the National Center for Youth Law, called at the time "psychiatric violence." In an article published in 1974, Opton identifies psychiatrists as central actors in the perpetration of psychiatric violence in prisons. He analyzes their actions and intentions in the context of three social roles: compliant accomplice, naive dupe, and pressured subordinate. As compliant accomplices, psychiatrists complacently permit prison administrators to use their clinical authority in service of punitive ends. As naive dupes, psychiatrists participate in psychiatric violence but "fail to see the plainly visible punitive use to which they are being put."[67] As pressured subordinates, psychiatrists enable the punitive misuse of their authority reluctantly, but they do not challenge that misuse.

For Opton, the distinction between treatment and punishment is specious, thus an ethical context is created in which a whole range of practices, from psychotropic drugging to psychosurgery, become morally permissible under the aegis of medical authority; the fundamental difference between treatment and punishment lies in the intent of the actor.[68] He writes: "An examination of the record of psychiatric treatment in prisons will show that prison psychiatrists are, in general, first and foremost functionaries in the disciplinary power structure of prison bureaucracy. Their interests are as adverse to the welfare of the prisoners as are those of the prison keepers."[69] From a constitutional standpoint, Opton argues that psychiatric treatments ought to be subjected to the same legal and ethical review applied to punishments.

Opton is one among many commentators, including prisoners themselves, who have drawn an analogy between psychotropic drugs and shackles.[70] "To immobilize a person against his will with drugs," he argues, "is violence for the same reasons that chaining a person to the wall with shackles is violence."[71] Unlike shackling, however, drugging causes permanent damage to the body and can be carried out inconspicuously on a large scale. Opton concludes that, put plainly, "most drugging is for the purpose of control, for keeping prisoners docile and quiet."[72] He quotes a former prisoner, who told him in an interview, "If you speak out, say things they don't like, if you're a leader, you know— it's an unspoken threat: they'll put you on Prolixin."[73] In a 1977 review of the principle of informed consent inside prisons and mental hospitals as it pertains to psychotropic drugging, law professor Richard Singer concludes, "Even discounting for paranoia, the nagging feeling remains, often because of the intense secrecy imposed on activities behind the walls and bars, that there is more truth to these rumors than we would wish to know."[74]

ANALYZING THE SILENCES

Throughout this book, I employ historical and comparative analyses of archival, scientific, and policy documents to chronicle meaning making in the social, medical, and ethical dimensions of psychotropics.[75] I argue that practices of knowledge production about psychotropic drugging make it exceedingly difficult to assess how drugging is used to uphold the U.S. carceral state. The coercive ways in which psychotropics serve to manufacture prisoners' silence are hidden behind practices of state secrecy, medical complicity, and corporate profiteering that result from and protect policies of mass confinement. Judging only by what I present in this book, it might seem as if we know quite a lot about psychotropic drugs in the U.S. carceral state, but knowing some things is different from knowing the right things.

I position silence as a way of talking about the effects of psychotropics on the brains and bodies of people living in the U.S. carceral state. Psychotropics transform the silencing function of custodial institutions by manufacturing a new kind of interior silence within the spirits/souls/psyches of individuals. Using psychotropics to act on a person's psychic spirit requires that state agents (i.e., administrators, guards, medical providers, officers) treat the spirit as if it is a material thing that can be forced into silence. People living within the carceral state are not literally dead (yet) or missing; rather, they are experiencing a kind of "spirit murder," which legal scholar Patricia Williams defines as "disregard for others whose lives qualitatively depend on our regard."[76] This spirit murder takes places, at least in part, through the unquestioned and largely unregulated use of psychotropics. The experience of spirit murder fosters a violent separation of human material existence from the spirit/soul/psyche, thus creating a new form of material and psychic existence. It is tempting to circumscribe materiality in such a way as to exclude the spirit life in favor of an understanding of life that is anchored in a hard, fleshy, and thus material, body.

I also use silence as a way of tracing the production of knowledge about psychotropics as part of a form of statecraft that generates mass confinement. This book is concerned with what we know as well as what we don't know about psychotropic use, and why we don't know what we don't know. In the chapters that follow, I raise questions about the government's practices of secrecy when it comes to the state-sanctioned distribution of psychotropics to confined people.[77] Questions of who produces knowledge and what they intend to do with that knowledge are central to the sociology of knowledge. When it comes to psychotropics, there are some things we can know and others we cannot know. Practices of knowledge production are dictated by the kinds of things that institutions of power want to know—governments possess unique means of producing social knowledge about the elements of society that interest them. Governments also possess the means to not produce knowledge about society and actively structure which kinds of knowledge become known to the public. Governments use social knowledge in strategic campaigns to shape public opinion, govern social behavior, and produce certain kinds of subjectivities and identities.

This book also excavates the troubling silence of scientific and official knowledge about institutional uses of psychotropic drugs. Do we know enough about what these drugs are doing to people to draw firm conclusions about their role in upholding mass confinement in the United States? The lack of knowledge about prisons' practices of psychotropic distribution serves to suppress knowledge about the utter failure of prisons and other confinement institutions to provide large numbers of psychically traumatized people with the humane and medically sound mental health care to which they are constitutionally and humanely entitled. Because scientists and prison administrators do not systematically evaluate psychotropic distribution practices in prisons and publish their information *publicly,* we do not know whether these practices result in improved psychiatric outcomes for prisoners or create new harms. Critics' claims that psychotropics are widely used to silence prisoners cannot readily be evaluated because no systematic knowledge exists regarding the extent and nature of the practice of administering psychotropics. Given these drugs' centrality to mental health care in prisons, surprisingly little is known about how frequently they are distributed, their biological effects on prisoners' brains and bodies, and what they might mean as biotechnologies that serve diverse social, medical, and political aims. Paradoxically, an extensive body of knowledge about psychotropics is available in the mainstream biomedical research literature produced in noninstitutionalized free society. So why is there silence about the use of psychotropics in prisons specifically?

The reason is that silence is central to the meaning and practices of subordination.[78] The U.S. carceral state requires dehumanizing forms of political ideology that can justify the legalized disappearance of millions of people and the suppression of social movements that actively oppose it. Silencing groups is a direct mechanism for achieving oppression and also an indirect means of suppressing opposition to that oppression. People living under oppressive social conditions are actively silenced through violent acts of murder and genocide, imprisonment and internment. Additionally, groups' oppositional voices are contained through marginalization and exclusion from media landscapes, communicative exchanges, and scholarly conversations. As Paulo Freire notes: "More and more, the oppressors are using science and technology as unquestionably powerful instruments for their purpose: the maintenance of the oppressive order through manipulation and repression. The oppressed, as objects, as 'things,' have no purposes except those their oppressors prescribe for them."[79] The transformation of people into "things" makes them vulnerable to horrible kinds of violence.[80]

To interpret this vulnerability to violence, I draw on two frameworks for understanding the social power involved in the use of psychotropics within the U.S. carceral state: biopower and necropower. Philosopher Michel Foucault used the framework of biopower, or biopolitics, to analyze social practices that target the biological processes of living organisms and entire species of organisms in the name of improving their health.[81] Biopower involves the production of biomedical knowledge about the health of organisms and the use of that knowledge to create social structures (e.g., public health agencies and health laws) that act on the health of the population of organisms as a whole. This new combination of science and social regulation began in the mid- to late 1800s, as European nation-states developed new strategies for increasing their national strength and political power. Foucault argued that the conduct of war, in which a nation exercised its right to kill its enemies, both foreign and domestic, was central to the power of government. During the transition to biopower, however, governments began to do something different to build national strength. European nation-states started producing their own scientific knowledge about the health of their populations through surveys, implementing new forms of social medicine designed to improve the health of their populations, and monitoring the labor force conditions of their populations, all in service of strengthening themselves through the mechanism of health.

In the framework of biopower, I view psychotropics as legitimate medical therapies that are more or less effective in managing the symptoms associated with psychiatric and emotional disorders. Psychotropics extend the power of biomedical psychiatry over the neurochemical terrain of the brain. Psychotropics are supposed to control patients' symptoms under the assumption that such symptoms are behavioral and cognitive expressions of underlying biochemical processes in the brain. With no discernible mental health infrastructure for the most impaired citizens and the impossibly high cost of talk therapy, U.S. citizens have had few options for mental health care beyond psychotropics. Psychotropics are prescribed for people in the name of improving their mental health. In this context, the distribution of psychotropics, however excessive or unregulated it might be in practice, is always theoretically legitimate and rational in the context of high levels of serious mental illness and trauma among captive populations. I take the position that one of the major limitations of the existing research on psychotropic use in institutions is that such use is always embedded within the context of attempts to *improve* mental health—that is, within the context of biopower.

While this interpretation of social power as biopolitical may justify the distribution of what may ultimately be billions of doses of psychotropics annually to persons living and dying within institutions, I question whether all that drugging is really done in the name of health. If we confine our view of the production of scientific knowledge about psychotropics and their distribution to what we can see through a biopolitical lens, we miss how psychotropics might be used to silence people, or worse. While the rhetoric of help, care, and mental health may reasonably justify the distribution of psychotropics to populations living in the U.S. carceral state, this meaning of psychotropics obscures their great potential as tools of social power that are all about destruction. What is the boundary between benevolent medicine and malevolent drugging? Psychiatric treatment involving psychotropics is always going to involve a measure of control, regardless of whether the intention is to heal or simply to pacify.

So, in this book I also turn to an alternative framework called necropower, or necropolitics, to explore these darker interpretations of psychotropic drugging. Social theorist Achille Mbembe has proposed necropower as a kind of philosophical corrective to Foucault's framework of biopower and its failure to account for social power that was, in fact, really still focused on killing the enemies of European nation-states. Viewing power through the historical contexts of European transnational slavery and colonialism, Mbembe argues that necropower is "the generalized instrumentalization of human existence and the material destruction of human bodies and populations."[82] In contrast to biopower, which functions through laws and other social regulations, necropower operates within what political theorist Giorgio Agamben calls "a state of exception"—a space outside the law in which murder can be carried out without regard for legal prohibitions against execution or assertions about individual rights under law.[83] In the context of necropower, governments target particular human social groups for death, define those groups as enemies, herd them into isolated territories with no viable social infrastructure, and use overwhelming technological force to kill them. Necropolitics creates what Mbembe calls death worlds, a "new and unique form of social existence in which vast populations are subjected to conditions of life conferring upon them the status of the living dead."[84]

Accordingly, through the framework of necropower, psychotropics are distributed to people in the name of producing mass psychic death. Here, the provision of psychotropics is potentially unethical, medically illegitimate, and unconstitutional. In other words, psychotropics are used to destroy psychic lives—the psychic lives of people who have already been socially sequestered for eventual disposal in places like prisons, people who have been socially abandoned. If the purpose of custody is to confine and ultimately eliminate unwanted social groups, psychotropics can be quite useful toward those evil ends.

These two frameworks also position the role of knowledge very differently. In stark contrast to the role that the production of scientific knowledge plays in shaping the biopolitics of a society, the production of epistemic silence, or willful ignorance, shapes the necropolitics of a society. These contrasting approaches to social power are also helpful in the evaluation of scientific, moral, and legal claims about the legitimacy or illegitimacy of medical practices. Determining whether a particular medical practice is understood as legitimate (because it promotes life and good health) or illegitimate (because it accelerates death and suffering) is contingent on the form of legal discourse that justifies the enactment of the practice itself. The conceptual boundary between legitimate and illegitimate practices is, like the theoretical contiguity of biopower and necropower, porous and indeterminate. The question should not be whether practices are legitimate or illegitimate, but rather how social power functions to obliterate any meaningful distinction between normal medicine and abnormal killing. As rates of psychotropic use have increased inside the U.S. carceral state, they have also steadily increased in so-called free society, making it more difficult to interpret what it means to be held captive in the first place.

In the first two chapters that follow, I explore the contrasting relationships between biomedical knowledge and bureaucratic information specifically within the prison system. In chapter 1, "Climbing the Walls," I examine what government surveys can tell us about prison pharmacoepidemiology, a scientific practice and knowledge that does not exist in a meaningful way for the purposes of evaluating government malfeasance. This science does not exist because it lacks an enduring institutional apparatus for collecting data. By detailing all of the major administrative surveys and institutional censuses concerning prescription drug use in prisons, this chapter outlines the scope of what prison pharmacoepidemiology can tell us, and what it cannot tell us, about the use of psychotropics among captive populations. As we will see, these limits foreclose attempts to answer many pressing questions about the use of psychotropics in prison and jail settings—a foreclosure that creates psychotropic ignorance.

In light of the built-in scientific limitations circumscribed by prison surveys and censuses, it has become increasingly difficult, if not entirely impossible, to determine the precise extent to which prisons are using psychotropics for any reason whatsoever, to say nothing of whether or not they are using them to control or silence prisoners. If there is one institution that should be able to provide the data needed to evaluate the claim that American prisons are systematically misusing psychotropics, it would be the prison pharmacy. In chapter 2, "The Pharmacy Prison," I analyze the key findings of government audits of prison pharmacies in order to understand both how these pharmacies operate as major conduits for drugs, especially psychotropics, and how they represent a fiscal and management crisis for prisons. The performance audits represent an innovative form of evidence, given the auditors' full statutory access to the prison pharmacies, prison policies, prisoner health records, institutional memory, and prison officials themselves. In many jurisdictions, government officials have required that teams of auditors examine prison policies, processes, and expenditures in order to determine whether money can be saved. Prison pharmacies have been found to be plagued by management problems, including poor record keeping and inventory systems, inadequate drug formularies, lack of space and well-trained personnel, and insufficient oversight.

In the next three chapters, I analyze legal and civic controversies involving psychotropics that bring psychiatry, prisoners' rights, and the police powers of the state into political contestation. Between 1941 and 1976, American prisoners made up the vast majority of research subjects for phase 1 and 2 clinical drug trials conducted in the United States (the four-phase clinical trial system began in 1962). Drug testing in prisons also became linked to citizenship in ways that validated white prisoners' sense of patriotism. In chapter 3, "Experimental Patriots," I analyze how pharmaceutical companies positioned prisoners' participation in drug tests as an altruistic act of patriotism and exercise of citizenship in order to justify ongoing drug testing regimes. In volunteering to be subjects in drug studies, white male prisoners were capable of becoming moral actors and better citizens. These "experimental patriots" also embodied a discourse of ethics, justice, and citizenship that aimed to justify the ongoing use of prisoners as drug test subjects. Through their participation, white prisoners were able to enact their citizenships in ways that were denied to black prisoners. Black prisoners' lesser participation was linked to their lesser status as citizens; they could not be real patriots who were willing to sacrifice their brains and bodies for the sake of the nation. Perhaps the whiteness of the prisoners used as subjects enabled the effort to construct the testing regimes as patriotic, as medical trials that, if carried out without further government regulation, would strengthen the nation by speeding up technoscientific progress and shoring up U.S. hegemony.

In chapter 4, I relate a series of stories within what I call "psychic states of emergency"—institutional crises that justify custodial power to hold bodies and, within those bodies, use psychotropics to transform brains for the purpose of managing vulnerable populations. States of emergency work by positioning brains and bodies on a thin boundary between therapeutic medical practice, in which people can choose to participate freely, and coercive state violence, which people cannot legally refuse. This chapter addresses populations other than prisoners who are also relegated to confinement—for wildly different kinds of reasons but with tragically similar outcomes. Psychotropics are increasingly distributed to active-duty soldiers, elders living in nursing homes and assisted care facilities, and children living under the aegis of the foster care system. Here, I extend the discussion beyond the confines of the carceral within state and federal prisons. While psychotropics may have helped to solve one institutional problem by enabling the closure of state mental hospitals and stabilizing the mental health of communities, today they are creating new problems of institutional abuse, neglect, and psychiatric harm.

While custodial institutions like prisons and state mental hospitals and asylums have long histories of experimental behavioral modification programs, psychotropics are used to enact violence on populations that are otherwise defined as dangerous. In chapter 5, "There Are Dark Days Ahead," I interpret psychotropics as neurochemical weapons that are deployed in extraordinary legal circumstances. In privately run federal detention centers, Immigration and Customs Enforcement (ICE) has been accused of forcibly administering psychotropics to civil detainees awaiting trial and deportation for immigration violations. In war-zone prisons in Iraq and Afghanistan, and at the Guantánamo Bay detention camp, the U.S. Department of Defense has, by its own admission, forcibly administered psychotropics to detainees prior to deportation and during marathon interrogation sessions; it has also used "chemical restraints" to manage threatening detainees. Elsewhere, high-dose antidepressants are being used to suppress the sexual desires of convicted sex offenders. By linking the use of psychotropics across these populations—undocumented immigrants, enemy combatants, and convicted sex offenders—I make the case that psychotropics have become indispensable to broader national security practices like border enforcement, international militarized conflict, and the prevention of sexual violence. Also in this chapter, I discuss the case of George Zimmerman, who, on the night he killed Trayvon Martin, had several psychotropics in his body—Restoril, Librax, and Adderall. Media reports suggested that Zimmerman had a history of violent behavior and that Zimmerman's father intervened on his behalf with the Sanford, Florida, police because of his son's history of psychiatric disturbances. Surprisingly, the prosecution and the news media downplayed Zimmerman's history of mental health problems and psychotropic use, which was potentially important to his state of mind. I situate Zimmerman's story within the context of biomedical research to examine the relationships among psychotropics, mental health, and gun violence.

In my Conclusion, "Overdose," I respond to the major counterfactual question in this book: Is it possible for the U.S. carceral state to exist in its current form without psychotropics? Like any good counterfactual, this question cannot be answered directly. But I think the answer is no. To make sense of this brutal counterfactual, I discuss the significance of psychotropics for existing institutionalized power arrangements that converge around the mental health of vulnerable groups and the theoretical ideas that draw attention to the problematic relationships between global pharmaceutical firms and the institutions of state and pharmaceutical capitalism that govern captive America. The current legal, scientific, and cultural classification of psychotropic drugs as therapeutic medicines requires revision in light of the ways that psychotropics are used to create new forms of social, psychic, and sexual death.

ONE

CLIMBING THE WALLS

A Survey of Psychotropic Ignorance

The defining architectural features of the prison are the walls—the real physical boundaries that separate the inside from the outside. Obviously, this closure captures the people who live and work in the prison; people do not flow freely across those physical boundaries. The doors remain locked, the walls are nearly impenetrable. Not so obviously, this closure also walls off information about what takes place on the inside. The prison is closed off not only to people but also to data, which have a hard time making their way into and out of the prison. The first problem I encountered when I began my research into the use of psychotropics in prison was finding out exactly what government-collected information was available on the topic. Cursory searches of both the scientific literature and government publications pointed me to an exceptionally narrow body of knowledge that reveals some of what we can know and, more important, what we cannot know about the use of psychotropics in prisons.

Administrative surveys of prisoners and institutional censuses are the central means by which we might know things about psychotropic use during incarceration. What they can tell us about these practices is limited, however—so limited that it might be said to qualify as a kind of nonknowledge, willful ignorance, or a front for malicious state secrecy.[1] It is not just that we don't know much about psychotropic drug use in prisons, it is that few procedures are in place to enable the collection of this information at all. Our knowledge is hampered by built-in limits to what can be known. I have examined all of the major population-based surveys of prescription drug use in prisons, and in this chapter I outline the scope of what prison pharmacoepidemiology can and cannot tell us about psychotropic use among imprisoned populations. Official government knowledge flows directly from the mechanisms of data collection that the government deploys. What the government knows is directly linked to the questions it asks. If the government does not ask certain questions, that leaves us in the dark.

The specific science that remains in the dark is pharmacoepidemiology, the study of the use and effects of drugs in populations.[2] This combination of pharmacology (the science of drugs and their effects on the body) and epidemiology (the science of population health) applies the theories and methods of epidemiology to the study of the distribution and effects of drugs in populations after the drugs' approval by the U.S. Food and Drug Administration (FDA). This science has its origins in the early twentieth century, when the nascent pharmaceutical industry experienced systemic problems with the safety of its products, leading to passage of the Pure Food and Drug Act of 1903. In 1961, pharmacoepidemiology experienced a seminal moment and began to play an important role in the U.S. drug regulatory process after the widely prescribed drug thalidomide, a sleeping aid marketed as safe for pregnant women, led to the births of thousands of babies worldwide with malformed limbs. This tragic episode spurred the development of the FDA's four-phase clinical trial process, in which drugs are subjected to scientific scrutiny before they can be sold to the general public.[3] (Relatedly, in chapter 3, I discuss the pivotal role that prisons and prisoners played in the unfolding of clinical drug trials in the United States.)

In addition to clinical trials, which are supposed to catch unsafe or ineffective drugs before they can go on the market, a parallel system has been established to monitor the safety of drugs after they have been approved for use in the general population. One key mechanism of this system is the FDA Adverse Event Reporting System (FAERS), which collects voluntary reports on "adverse events" and "medication errors" from health professionals, consumers, and drug companies.[4] Using the interactive Public Dashboard tool available on the FDA's website, members of the public can enter the names of drugs and see detailed and historical information about adverse events related to those drugs.[5] This system, the very best source of public information about adverse drug events that the U.S. government has to offer, is not perfect; as the FDA website notes, the Public Dashboard tool "cannot be used to calculate the incidence of an adverse event or medication error in the U.S. population."[6] In 2007, the FDA added another system called Postmarket Drug and Biologic Safety Evaluations, which monitors the safety of drugs eighteen months after their FDA approval or after they have been used by ten thousand people.[7]

Beyond these formal federal monitoring systems, numerous population health surveys collect data on psychotropic drug use in the general U.S. population.[8] A growing body of research has analyzed sociological patterns in access to mental health services and psychotropic use in the noninstitutionalized U.S. population.[9] Ryne Paulose-Ram and colleagues used nationally representative data from the National Health and Nutrition Examination Survey for the years 1988–91 to analyze psychotropic drug use and found that women used psychotropics at nearly twice the rate of men (4.6 percent versus 7.5 percent); they also found that African Americans and Mexican Americans self-reported lower use than did non-Hispanic whites (5.1 percent, 4.5 percent, and 6.6 percent, respectively).[10] Studies of prescribing patterns for psychotropics suggest that members of racial and ethnic minority groups are less likely than whites to receive these drugs for a range of psychiatric diagnoses. Using 1992–2000 data from more than 5,000 patient visits recorded in the National Ambulatory Medical Care Survey and the National Hospital Ambulatory Care Medical Survey, Gail Daumit and her colleagues found that African Americans and Hispanics were less likely than whites to receive atypical antipsychotics, drugs that produce more side effects and are generally considered less effective than other drugs in managing psychotic disorders.[11] This finding was supported by the results of a smaller, local study of 1,245 psychiatric patients.[12] Other studies have found that African Americans and Hispanics with depression are less likely than whites with depression to receive pharmacotherapy, and the same racialized pattern holds true for anxiety disorders and among veterans with bipolar disorder.[13]

It is important to note that institutionalized populations are regularly excluded from large-scale population health surveys, and they are definitely not included in large-scale studies of the generalized effects of prescription drugs. There is so much we do not know, and cannot know, about psychotropic drug use in prisons because of the particular ways in which the government has designed health surveys of prisoners and prison health care practices, both historically and today. Despite the large numbers of prisoners with mental health problems, it is impossible to know whether the patterns of psychotropic use in U.S. prisons are consistent with those in noninstitutionalized contexts (see chapter 4 for discussion of other institutionalized populations). The ignorance that permeates prison pharmacoepidemiology contrasts with the proliferation of knowledge about psychotropics in so-called free society.

QUANTIFYING PSYCHOTROPICS IN PRISONS

The U.S. prison system is not a unified, coherent thing. Rather, it is made up of many individual systems at different jurisdictional levels: city/county, state, federal, military, extralegal. This institutional heterogeneity presents a challenge to researchers and advocates who are trying to make sense of patterns of practice across and within systems. For the purposes of this chapter, I have set aside the array of small-scale studies conducted ad hoc by researchers in particular jurisdictions, examining an individual jail, for instance, or one state-level department of corrections. These local studies, which are relatively small in number, do provide important information about localized practices in particular places at particular moments in time. The Texas system is a good example. In the late 1990s, Jacques Baillargeon and colleagues conducted a pair of studies on prescribing patterns within the Texas prison system, one focused on antidepressants and the other on antipsychotics.[14] They found that among Texas prisoners with formal diagnoses of depressive disorders, black and Latino prisoners were less likely than whites to be placed on selective serotonin reuptake inhibitors and more likely not to be prescribed any antidepressant treatment. Black prisoners were more likely than either Hispanics or whites to be prescribed tricyclic antidepressants.[15] I imagine that this analysis was possible because the UT Medical System, for which Baillargeon and his colleagues worked, was the primary provider of medical care in the Texas prison system. The researchers were able to collect data on Texas prisoners' psychotropic use through the medical records system shared by the UT Medical System and the prisons.

Such local studies may be both interesting and important, but they do not contribute much to the goal of constructing an empirical bird's-eye view of the U.S. prison system as a whole that will allow us to evaluate claims about the use of psychotropics at the levels of all U.S. prisoners and across all U.S. prison institutions. A recent international meta-analysis found that issues of polypharmacy (the use of more than one drug at the same time), high and long-term dosing, and lack of documentation and monitoring are important in prison contexts; unfortunately, the authors identify only two articles reporting on research conducted within U.S. systems, neither of which actually documents system-wide use of psychotropics.[16] One of the articles reports on individual cases of quetiapine abuse in Ohio prison facilities, and the other discusses the metabolic syndrome monitoring system used by the New Jersey Department of Corrections and focuses on prisoners taking second-generation antipsychotics.[17]

If we had comprehensive and consistent information, going back decades, on the numbers of prisoners who have been administered psychotropics and for what reasons, that would be incredibly valuable for the science of pharmacoepidemiology. We do not have such information, however. First of all, the federal government has been collecting any form of nationally representative data about prisoners' health only since 1974; before then, no systematic effort was made to collect any health information on prisoners. It would be hard to prove, but my guess is that the collection of prisoner health data began in response to the prisoner revolt and subsequent massacre at Attica Correctional Facility in 1971, the same year that the National Prisoner Statistics Program was transferred to the Bureau of Justice Statistics from the Federal Bureau of Prisons. The program started collecting statistical data each year on federal and state prisons back in 1926, although episodic raw counts of U.S. prisoners had been made as early as the 1850 census.[18] Figure 1 lists the major administrative surveys of prisoners and institutional prison censuses that ask any questions about psychotropic use during incarceration. In the next section, I explore the questions these instruments ask in order to bring to light what they can tell us about psychotropic use in U.S. prisons and jails.

ADMINISTRATIVE SURVEYS OF PRISONERS

Prisoners are seldom asked whether they have been prescribed or have taken psychotropic drugs during their period of incarceration, and because such queries were not included in multiple survey years over time, cross-sectional analysis is difficult, and historical analysis is impossible. Surveys have inconsistently assessed prisoners' mental health status over time, complicating any effort to pose questions about the appropriateness of reported psychotropic use as a therapy for diagnosed psychiatric illness or reported psychological distress. Relatedly, surveys have conflated prisoners who report taking psychotropics during incarceration with prisoners who have psychiatric diagnoses, as if everyone who takes such drugs in prison is, by definition, mentally ill.

The Survey of Inmates in State Correctional Facilities (SISCF), a

Name of Survey	Survey Years
Survey of Inmates in State Correctional Facilities	1974, 1979, 1986, 1991, 1997
Survey of Inmates in Federal Correctional Facilities	1991, 1997
Survey of Inmates in State and Federal Correctional Facilities	2004
Survey of Prison Inmates	2016
Survey of Inmates in Local Jails	1972, 1978, 1983, 1989, 1992, 1996, 2002
National Inmate Survey	2007, 2008–9, 2011–12
Census of State and Federal Adult Correctional Facilities	1974, 1979, 1984, 1990, 1995, 2000, 2005
National Survey of Prison Health Care	2011

FIGURE 1. Prisoner administrative surveys and institutional censuses.

nationally representative survey of inmates housed in state prisons within all U.S. states, began collecting data on state prisoners in 1974 and continued every five years. In 2004, it was combined with the Survey of Inmates in Federal Correctional Facilities (SIFCF) to form the Survey of Inmates in State and Federal Correctional Facilities (SISFCF), which was later renamed the Survey of Prison Inmates. Each wave of the SISCF was structured to link the probability for selection of any inmates to the sizes of the facilities where they were incarcerated. In the first stage of the study design, statisticians created independent sampling frames for male and female prisons and then stratified prisons by census region and facility type (i.e., confinement versus community corrections) within each frame. In 1991, an additional sampling frame was added for security level of the facility (maximum, medium, minimum). In the second stage, prison officials provided rosters to census officials who then selected inmates randomly according to predetermined targets established by the Bureau of Justice Statistics.[19] Interviewers from the U.S. Census Bureau conducted face-to-face interviews with consenting inmates in their facilities. Inmate participation was voluntary, and prisoners' individual responses to survey questions were confidential and anonymous.

With each successive wave of the survey, questions about psychotropic use changed in important ways, making cross-wave comparisons nearly impossible. First, the key question of whether the inmate was currently taking a psychotropic drug was asked of the entire sample of inmates only in 1979, 1986, and 1991, and the wording and clarifying follow-up questions changed over time. In 1979, prisoners were asked a series of questions. First, they were asked if they were currently taking any medications. If they said yes, they were then asked to identify the names of up to three medications they were currently taking. In 1986, prisoners were asked if they were currently taking medications for "mental problems," and in 1991, they were asked if they had taken medications for emotional or mental problems since they had been admitted to prison. In 1986 and 1991, inmates were not asked the follow-up question about their current medication use. To my knowledge, official government reports have not referenced these data about mental health care in state prisons, in part because of these differences in the questionnaires over time.

The 1997 and 2004 waves of the SISCF did ask whether inmates were taking psychotropic drugs during their incarceration; rather, only inmates who had *ever* taken psychotropic drugs prior to their imprisonment were asked this question. In 1999, the Bureau of Justice Statistics published a report titled *Mental Health and Treatment of Inmates and Probationers* based on data from the 1997 SISCF, the 1996 Survey of Inmates in Local Jails, and the 1995 Survey of Adults on Probation. For the purposes of the analysis, state inmates were defined as having a mental illness if they had "a current mental or emotional condition" or had experienced "an overnight stay in a mental hospital or treatment program."[20] Given these criteria, 16.2 percent of state prison inmates reported mental illness. From this survey, we know that in 1997, 60 percent of mentally ill prisoners received some form of mental health treatment; 50 percent of those who received any treatment received psychotropics.[21] By contrast, 44 percent had received counseling or therapy and 24 percent had been hospitalized overnight in a mental hospital. The way in which these questions are nested, and the fact that they are not asked of every state inmate, really limits what we know about drugging practices in state prisons. In 1996, according to data from the Survey of Inmates in Local Jails, 41 percent of mentally ill inmates received some form of mental health treatment—only 34 percent of them were given psychotropics. This survey has been conducted seven times, in 1972, 1978, 1983, 1989, 1992, 1996, and 2002. But 1996 was the only survey year in which a question about psychotropic use during incarceration was asked.

In 2004, as noted above, the SISCF and SIFCF were conducted at the same time, together becoming the Survey of Inmates in State and Federal Correctional Facilities. The 2004 wave asked a series of questions about prisoner mental health and included, for the first time, a modified structural clinical interview focused on psychiatric symptoms for major depression, mania, and psychosis as specified in the fourth edition of the *Diagnostic and Statistical Manual of Mental Disorders*.[22] The survey also asked prisoners if they were taking a prescription psychotropic medication *in the year prior to* their incarceration; 18 percent of state prisoners, 14.4 percent of jail inmates, and 10.3 percent of federal prisoners answered yes.[23] A secondary analysis of data from the 2004 SISFCF and the 2002 Survey of Inmates in Local Jails found that 69.1 percent of federal prisoners, 68.6 percent of state prisoners, and 45.5 percent of jail inmates *with diagnosed disorders* had taken psychotropics during their incarceration.[24] Taken together, these data also show that at each level of duration of incarceration, from jail detention to long-term imprisonment, prisoners are prescribed psychotropics more often than they receive other mental health treatments.[25]

In 2016, the SISFCF was renamed the Survey of Prison Inmates. In that survey year, the following sequence of questions about psychotropic drug use was introduced:

> At the time of [your offense], were you taking prescription medicine for any problem you were having with your emotions, nerves, or mental health?

> Since you were admitted to prison, have you taken prescription medicine for any problem you were having with your emotions, nerves, or mental health?

If the respondent answered yes to the second question, he or she was then asked:

> Are you *currently* taking prescription medicine for any problem with your emotions, nerves, or mental health?

All respondents, regardless of their prior mental health diagnoses, were asked this sequence of questions, an improvement over previous surveys, because it enables the evaluation of psychotropic use within prisons across nationally representative populations of state and federal inmates. However, because the questions are new, the data gathered using them can be analyzed only for the 2016 survey year so far, and these data are not yet publicly available.

The National Inmate Survey is a collaborative survey of a 10 percent sample of correctional facilities that includes a minimum of one prison and one jail in each U.S. state. Conducted by the Research Triangle Institute under contract with the Bureau of Justice Statistics, the National Inmate Survey is *the* survey mechanism for ensuring correctional institutions' compliance with the Prison Rape Elimination Act of 2003. The survey was first conducted in 2007, with additional waves following in 2008–9 and 2011–12. The 2011–12 wave was conducted in 233 state and federal prisons, 358 jails, and 15 special facilities (e.g., military, ICE, and Native American tribal facilities) between February 2011 and May 2012. In this wave, adult prisoners in federal and state prisons (but not the special facilities) were asked about their mental health histories and prescription psychotropic use since their incarceration. More than 100,000 prisoners and detainees participated in the survey. The 2007 and 2008–9 surveys did not ask about drug use. A report on the 2011–12 survey's findings was published in June 2017.[26]

In the survey, only prisoners who reported having diagnosed mental health problems prior to their incarceration were asked the following questions about psychotropic drugs and alternative mental health treatments:

Have you ever taken any prescription medicine for any problem you were having with your emotions, nerves, or mental health?

At the time of the offense for which you are currently serving time, were you taking prescription medicine for any problem you were having with your emotions, nerves, or mental health?

Since you were admitted to any facility to serve time on your current sentence, have you taken prescription medicine for any problem you were having with your emotions, nerves, or mental health?

Are you currently taking prescription medicine for any problem with your emotions, nerves, or mental health?

The survey then asked a detailed battery of questions about five categories of mental health problems: manic depression, bipolar disorder, or mania; depressive disorder; schizophrenia or psychotic disorder; post-traumatic stress disorder (PTSD) or anxiety disorder; and personality disorder. For each category, the following sequence of questions was asked:

> In the 30 days before you were admitted to this facility, were you taking any prescription medicine for your [mental health problem]?
>
> In the 30 days before you were admitted to any facility to serve time on your current sentence, were you taking any prescription medicine for your [mental health problem]?
>
> Since you were admitted to this facility, have you taken any prescription medicine for your [mental health problem]?
>
> Since you were admitted to any facility to serve time on your current sentence, have you taken any prescription medicine for your [mental health problem]?
>
> Think about when you were first told that you had [this mental health problem] after you were admitted to any facility to serve time on your current sentence. How soon after you were told did you start taking prescription medicine for your [mental health problem]?
>
> Are you currently taking prescription medicine for your [mental health problem]?

If the respondent answered no to the preceding question, this follow-up question was asked:

> Why aren't you currently taking prescription medicine for your [mental health problem]?

So, while the National Inmate Survey provides the most comprehensive data on psychotropic use among prisoners with mental health diagnoses to date, it is structured in such a way that it does not capture respondents who have not been diagnosed with mental health problems but are nevertheless prescribed psychotropics or forced to take them in prison. It also provides no information about inmates who did not take such drugs prior to incarceration but may be taking them now. On one hand, this narrow approach makes sense given the survey's focus on mental health care delivery—prison administrators want to know how well they are meeting the mental health needs of their inmates with acknowledged mental health problems. But on the other hand, the questions that are not being asked are the ones that might make it possible to tease out information about potential forced medication, overdosing, misdiagnoses, and prescribing errors.

INSTITUTIONAL CENSUSES OF PRISONS

While prisoner surveys provide useful but limited information about psychotropic use at the level of the prisoner, institutional censuses also shed light on the practice. In these censuses, prison officials themselves are queried about the policies and practices of their institutions. In 2000, the Census of State and Federal Adult Correctional Facilities included all 84 federal facilities, 1,320 state facilities, and 264 private facilities in operation on June 30, 2000.[27] Across the years this census has been conducted—1974, 1979, 1984, 1990, 1995, 2000, and 2005—only the 1979, 1984, and 2000 iterations have asked about psychotropics, and the question was different each time:

In 1979: "How many prisoners are receiving prescription medication for mental or emotional stress, anxiety, or depression?"

In 1984: "How many residents/inmates are receiving psychotropic medications (such as Thorazine and Stelazine)?"

In 2000: "Of all inmates confined in your facility on June 30, 2000, how many were receiving psychotropic medications (drugs having a mind-altering effect, e.g., antidepressants, stimulants, sedatives, tranquilizers, and other anti-psychotic drugs?)"

From the 2000 census, we know that, as a matter of policy, 73 percent of state prisons distributed psychotropics to prisoners and 71 percent provided therapy or counseling, although only 65 percent conducted psychiatric assessments. As a matter of practice, 10 percent of all state inmates were receiving psychotropics; 13 percent were in therapy or counseling. That amounts to 114,400 state prisoners receiving psychotropics in 2000. In five states at least 20 percent of prisoners were receiving psychotropics: Hawaii, Maine, Montana, Nebraska, and Oregon. In Alabama, Arkansas, and Michigan, in contrast, less than 5 percent of prisoners were taking such drugs. The California Medical Facility at Vacaville stands out among all state prisons in that year: 42 percent of the 3,070 inmates were taking psychotropics. Perhaps coincidentally, this facility was also the site of an extensive biomedical research program in the 1960s (see chapter 3).

From this census, we know that 95 percent of maximum-security prisons had policies concerning psychotropic distribution, compared to 88 percent of medium-security prisons and only 62 percent of minimum-security facilities. Additionally, the proportion of prisoners receiving psychotropics was higher in maximum-security (11 percent) than in medium- (10 percent) and minimum-security facilities (6 percent). More prisoners in public prisons than in private prisons took psychotropics (10 percent versus 7.7 percent). As far as I have been able to discern, this is the only time that an official report has mentioned the issue of psychotropic use in privately operated prisons. Prison size was also related to psychotropic policies: lower proportions of prisoners from large prisons (750 prisoners or more) took psychotropics compared with prisoners in smaller prisons (9.6 percent versus 10.4 percent).

The National Survey of Prison Health Care, conducted in 2011, was a onetime collaboration between the National Center for Health Statistics and the Bureau of Justice Statistics that asked prison medical officials about the provision and delivery of health care to prisoners.[28] The survey targeted all fifty state prison systems and all correctional institutions overseen by the Federal Bureau of Prisons. It asked respondents if the prisons where they worked conducted mental health assessments and whether they had contract agreements for pharmaceutical services, but it did not ask about the provision of psychotropics to prisoners. This is a remarkable omission for a survey that was supposed to focus on health care services, and a strange omission given the history of questioning that preceded it.

Equitable access to high-quality mental health treatment should be an important goal in U.S. prisons and jails, but more prison pharmacoepidemiology is necessary to document patterns of practice and inequity in the system. The fact that vast public resources are allocated to mental health treatment for incarcerated persons further justifies efforts toward closer scientific scrutiny of psychotropic drug distribution in U.S. prisons. This research should cover many aspects of psychotropic prescribing practices in prisons. No survey has ever asked prisoners if they were forcibly administered psychotropics or if they were prescribed psychotropics without first receiving psychiatric evaluation. We cannot know about psychotropic use among prisoners who have not been diagnosed with psychiatric disorders. We cannot know whether psychotropics have been used forcibly in cases of crisis intervention or in emergency psychiatric units. We cannot know about drug-specific uses within and across prison systems. We cannot document historical use trends that account for changes in prison population growth in relationship to patterns of mental illness. We cannot know anything about undocumented uses of psychotropics in any prison system.

To make this problem even more difficult, we cannot know any and all of these things within and across racialized and gendered groups of prisoners. It has long been known that men and people of color are disproportionately incarcerated in the United States; what is needed now is a better understanding of how race and gender structure the provision of health treatment among these vulnerable institutionalized populations.[29] Unfortunately, the research conducted on psychotropic drug use thus far has focused either on racial and ethnic minority groups or on specific gender groups, with no attention to the intersection of racial and gender structures. No study has documented or analyzed patterns of psychotropic drug use among state prisoners within specific race and gender groups. This narrow vision has led to a partial understanding of the mental health crisis among prisoners. A number of small-scale case studies suggest that women prisoners are more likely than their male counterparts to receive psychotropic drugs, but we have no idea how this difference looks when race and ethnicity are also considered.[30]

Surveys and censuses foreclose many pressing questions concerning the use of psychotropics in prisons. Why do these government instruments do such a relatively poor job of documenting psychotropic drug use in the prison system? Just as the prison itself is designed to keep people locked in, these instruments are designed to keep prying eyes out. The next chapter describes an effort to get up and over the walls of the prison to learn more about how prisons deliver prescription drugs.

THE PHARMACY PRISON

Auditing Prison Pharmaceutical Regimes

(with Renee M. Shelby)

In 1936, Charles L. Pickens, an administrative assistant within the U.S. Public Health Service stationed at the U.S. Penitentiary Hospital in Atlanta, Georgia, presented what he believed was the first paper given by a prison pharmacist before the American Pharmaceutical Association. In his remarks, Pickens suggested that working as a pharmacist inside a federal prison was a very interesting experience. "If Government regulations permitted my telling you a lot of inside stories of many of the country's most notorious criminals whom I have known and worked with during the last ten and a half years," Pickens opened up to the group, "I could hold your attention whether you were any wiser when I finished or not, but regulations prevent, so that is out of the picture."[1] The official story Pickens told was that in the prior year, 1935, there were 90,215 sick calls made in the Atlanta Penitentiary, leading to 32,467 prescriptions.[2] (A sick call represents an inmate's formal request for medical treatment.) He was responsible for mixing all of the chemical preparations and for hiring inmate support staff to work within the pharmacy; he also had to be part detective in order to prevent the diversion of drugs in the institution. Prison pharmacists, Pickens pointed out, do not face the same problems as commercial pharmacists:

> We do not have the financial worries of the retail pharmacy as all bills are paid by the Treasury Department. . . . We have no tax problems; no windows to keep dressed to encourage business *as we have all the business we want.* . . . We have no credit business, as the medicines and all other supplies are furnished gratis to any and all inmates requiring them.[3]

"We have all the business we want." That is, unlike the local CVS or Walgreens, the prison pharmacy has no need to drum up business, no need to sell sodas and cigarettes in order to increase sales—the bills are paid in full, and the queue of customers never ends. (Actually, retail pharmacies like CVS and Walgreens are in the prison pharmacy business, too, in that they provide ad hoc emergency pharmacy services when standard prison procurement systems break down.) Pickens made the prison pharmacy sound like a dream business. He ended his remarks with words that could have come from a promotional brochure for the prison as a tourist destination: "I would suggest that when you have the opportunity that you visit a Federal Penitentiary, for, after all, they are your prisons and we only work there."[4]

What kind of work actually takes place in a prison pharmacy? The prison pharmacy is the bureaucratic office that processes doctors' prescriptions, procures drugs, manages drug inventories, and distributes drugs to prisoners. If there is one institution that has the potential to contain the information needed to evaluate the claim that American prisons are systematically misusing psychotropics, it is the prison pharmacy. If administrative surveys and institutional censuses do not provide exhaustive accounts of the provision of psychotropics inside prison walls (as discussed in chapter 1), perhaps the prison pharmacy can provide that accounting. Imagine for a moment what an audit of a prison pharmacy might reveal under ideal circumstances. Assume that we want to know whether Prison Guard Brown has been using psych meds to keep Prisoner Johnson quiet and controlled. Assume that Prisoner Johnson has no diagnosed mental illness, a fact that we know because the prison conducts thorough and repeated psychiatric evaluations on all of its prisoners. Guard Brown will have needed to document each instance in which she has asked Dr. Smith to give a powerful antipsychotic drug to Prisoner Johnson—there would be a written record of each request. We could then look for documentation that any given request resulted in Dr. Smith's submission of a prescription for Prisoner Johnson to the prison pharmacy technician. And then we could look for any record that this technician filled the prescription in the modern pharmacy inventory system that the prison is required to maintain. We could link that process back to Prisoner Johnson by examining documentation in his medical records, which would show that he was administered antipsychotics, apparently for no justifiable medical reason. Let's take it one step further: we could aggregate other cases like

Prisoner Johnson's to reveal a pattern of medical mistreatment within that particular facility or across prisons. If such an audit process were possible, we would be able to answer questions about the medical abuse of psychotropics *definitively and empirically*. But this is an exercise in hypothetical fantasy.

Obviously, we cannot simply walk into a prison pharmacy and demand that it open up its medical records, inventory systems, and documented staff communications for critical scrutiny. But that is exactly what state and privately contracted auditors have done in many prisons under the force of law. Prison pharmacies across the country have been subjected to audit processes similar to the fictitious one I describe above. Because of the extraordinary amount of money prisons spend on psychotropic drugs, government officials have required that teams of state-sanctioned auditors examine prison pharmacy policies, processes, and expenditures. Their concern is with saving money, however, not with identifying medical abuses.

Because prison pharmacoepidemiology provides so little knowledge about prisoners' use of psychotropic drugs, in this chapter I use prison pharmacy audits as alternative sources of information. In the following pages, I synthesize information about prison pharmacy practices from thirty-one publicly available prison and jail pharmacy audits to describe how prisons operate as major conduits for prescription drugs. The audits cover the period from fiscal year 1999 through the end of calendar year 2014, and they span federal, state, and city/county jurisdictions (Figure 2 lists the year of publication, facility or system name, and jurisdiction of each of the audits reviewed). This historical period roughly corresponds to the time when selective serotonin reuptake inhibitors (SSRIs) and atypical antipsychotics were entering the pharmaceutical market. Each audit was conducted with a specific mandate for a particular jurisdiction, so the audit reports do not convey parallel information about pharmacy practices; generally, however, a set of themes and government preoccupations structure how such audits are organized and carried out.

While there are themes that cut across jurisdictions, I try to focus here on what these audits say about psychotropics. Prison pharmacy audits provide a unique angle of vision into the systems of knowledge production and accountability (or lack thereof) that influence prison pharmacy practices. Given the auditors' full and open access to prison pharmacy records as well as prison policies, prisoner health records,

Year of Publication	Facility/Department/System Name	Jurisdiction
2011	State Correctional Institution at Laurel Highlands	Pennsylvania
2013	State Correctional Institution at Graterford	Pennsylvania
2007	Corrections Department	New Mexico
2011	Corrections Department	New Mexico
2001	Department of Corrections	Wisconsin
2009	Department of Corrections	Wisconsin
2011	Department of Corrections	Michigan
2008	Department of Corrections	New Hampshire
2014	County Jail	Allegany County, New York
2005	Department of Corrections	Colorado
2009	Division of Prisons	North Carolina
2003	Department of Corrections	Georgia
2010	Department of Corrections and Rehabilitation	California
2006	Department of Corrections	Nevada
2013	Federal Bureau of Prisons	United States
2005	Federal Bureau of Prisons	United States
2007	County Adult Detention Center	Salt Lake County, Utah
2004	Department of Corrections and Rehabilitation	North Dakota
2007	Department of Corrections	Oklahoma
2011	Department of Corrections	Iowa
2013	Department of Corrections	Utah
2007	Department of Adult and Juvenile Detention	King County, Washington
2013	Department of Corrections	Vermont
2014	County Correctional Facility	Erie County, New York
2015a	Department of Corrections	Nebraska

Year of Publication	Facility/Department/System Name	Jurisdiction
2015b	Department of Corrections	Nebraska
2009	County Jail	Sacramento County, California
2014	County Jail	Washington County, Oregon
2009	Department of Corrections	Tennessee
2014	Division of Youth Corrections Facilities	Colorado
2014	Department of Corrections	Minnesota

FIGURE 2. Prison pharmacy audits.

institutional memory, and prison officials themselves, these audits represent a unique form of official knowledge about the institutional practices that govern psychotropics. The auditors had statutory authority to access any and all information relative to the mandate outlined by the state legislatures or federal authorities. They sampled and systematically reviewed prisoner medical records, interviewed prison staff, and accessed pharmacy inventory and expenditure records—virtually no information was considered to be outside the scope of their jurisdiction. The auditors then reported back to their governing bodies, basing their findings on all of the information available to them; these findings are a kind of evidentiary gold standard that outside academic researchers could only hope to achieve even under ideal circumstances in prison contexts. While the auditors did not necessarily ask the same kinds of questions that researchers or prisoners' advocates might ask, their unfettered access to and framing of the evidence of pharmacy practices and psychotropic distribution warrant critical scrutiny. Prison audit reports represent high-quality sources of information about what takes place inside prisons, and they are less subject than the work of outside researchers to possible criticisms about methodological weaknesses or political biases.

PRISON PHARMACEUTICAL REGIMES

Across the United States, prison pharmacies are situated within a web of public and private institutions that manage the prescribing, procurement, distribution, and disposal of pharmaceuticals. These pharmaceutical regimes feature clinical workers and medical practitioners (physicians, nurses, pharmacists), regulatory structures (laws, contracts, policies, procedures), information technologies (inventory and delivery systems), and, of course, the pharmaceuticals themselves. These regimes are configured within local, state, and national jurisdictional contexts across the thousands of individual prisons and jail systems within the United States. There are vast institutional differences across these systems, so it is not analytically useful to talk about *one kind* of prison pharmacy. But it is important to talk about all of these systems operating within coordinated networks of government, corporate, and professional medical institutions—prison pharmaceutical regimes.

One central node in this network is the Minnesota Multistate Contracting Alliance for Pharmacy (MMCAP). Established in 1985 through a cooperative agreement among several Minnesota state agencies, the University of Minnesota, and Ramsey and Hennepin Counties (which are home to the major metropolitan areas of the Twin Cities) and currently managed by the Materials Management Division of the state of Minnesota's Department of Administration, MMCAP is

> a free, voluntary group purchasing organization for government facilities that provide healthcare services. . . . MMCAP's membership extends across nearly every state in the nation, delivering volume buying power. Members receive access to a full range of pharmaceuticals and other healthcare products and services, such as medical supplies, influenza vaccine, dental supplies, drug testing, wholesaler invoice auditing, and returned goods processing.[5]

Strangely, as noted in an audit done by Minnesota's Office of the Legislative Auditor, the Minnesota Department of Corrections currently does not purchase its own pharmaceuticals through MMCAP, but rather through Corizon, its contracted health services vendor.[6] It may seem odd that the Minnesota Department of Corrections does not buy its drugs through this alliance within its home state, but, as we will see, this is not the only curious thing about prison pharmacies.

Using economies of scale, MMCAP enables governments to purchase bulk pharmaceuticals at lower prices. More than five thousand individual government facilities—including correctional facilities, psychiatric treatment facilities, student health services, public health services, nonfederal veterans' nursing homes, public hospitals, and veterinary clinics/hospitals—purchase their pharmaceuticals through MMCAP.

Collectively, MMCAP members purchase more than $1 billion worth of pharmaceuticals and other medical supplies each year. According to Brandon Sis, coordinator of the corrections branch of MMCAP's Clinical Pharmacy Program, as of June 9, 2017, 18 percent of MMCAP members were correctional institutions.[7] Given the overall membership number, that means that approximately nine hundred individual correctional institutions purchase pharmaceuticals through MMCAP.

According to its website, MMCAP provides governments "a voice" in its operations, helps facilitate careful contract management, and offers reduced costs for products and services, access to standardized formularies, procurement guidelines that meet state requirements, and, of course, customer service.[8] MMCAP contracts with three pharmaceutical wholesalers: AmerisourceBergen, Cardinal Health, and Morris & Dickson. These companies purchase pharmaceuticals directly from manufacturers and distribute them to individual facilities, which pay fees back to MMCAP for negotiating the deals; MMCAP's operations are financed by these fees. The three wholesalers are massive global companies on their own, and together they constitute a vast network for the distribution of pharmaceuticals to government institutions through MMCAP.

While hundreds of prisons procure pharmaceuticals through consortia like MMCAP, many correctional systems have turned to private pharmacy management companies, like Corizon and its pharmacy unit PharmaCorr, to run their pharmacies. Corizon operates in 301 individual facilities in twenty-two U.S. states.[9] PharmaCorr runs in-house pharmacies in Indiana and Oklahoma and mail-order pharmacy services in sixteen states.[10] Corizon was formed in 2011 through a merger between Prison Health Services and Correctional Medical Services and is owned by the large firm Valitas Health Services, which itself is majority owned by Beecken Petty O'Keefe, a private equity firm.[11] Companies like PharmaCorr, Diamond Pharmacy Services, Correctional Pharmacy Services, Correct Care Solutions, and Boswell Pharmacy Services also provide intermediary and direct services to prison systems.

The amount of public funds devoted to sustaining mass incarceration is truly breathtaking. Many taxpayer dollars are paid out to private companies like these, which deliver health-related goods and services within prison systems. Every dollar spent by the government for the health of prisoners is a dollar received by a private health corporation—

prisons, and the prisoners within them, represent an important node in the circuitry of biomedical capitalism. Providing prisoners with all of the commodities that cycle through their bodies, most notably food and drugs, is a really big business.[12] According to a 2014 report from the Pew Charitable Trusts and the MacArthur Foundation, in fiscal year 2011, the fifty states spent a total of approximately $7.7 billion on prison health care, an amount representing about one out of every five state dollars spent on imprisonment.[13] From 2007 to 2011, spending on pharmaceuticals accounted for 14 percent of total spending on prisons for the ten states that submitted comprehensive data to the researchers.[14] And prisons' pharmacy-related expenditures are increasing in many jurisdictions. Legislative changes are one factor driving up health care costs, as mandatory minimum sentencing and three-strikes laws keep prisoners incarcerated longer than ever before, leaving prisons to deal with the increased costs of caring for older prisoners. Prisons are constitutionally required to provide inmates with adequate health care, and failure to do so can leave states open to expensive lawsuits. For example, from 1996 to 2002 alone, the state of Washington spent more than $1.26 million on judgments and settlements as the result of claims of poor prison health care.[15]

In 2004, a report published by the Council of State Governments noted that "no national data exists on how much each state pays for inmate pharmaceutical products," and that is still true today.[16] A neoliberal form of economic rationality organizes decision making in the current prison pharmaceutical regime. This rationality is linked to a discourse and accompanying systems of accountability that take the form of the audit. Prison officials are constantly trying to find ways to reduce health care costs while not ignoring their legal obligation to provide adequate care. To save money, some prisons now demand copayments from prisoners for medical services; other cost-saving measures include improving efficiencies through the use of technologies such as telemedicine and automation of inventory systems, privatizing health care clinical labor, using formularies and more generic drugs, establishing effective disease prevention programs, and expanding early release of terminally ill and elderly patients.

High and increasing costs for prison health care have forced government officials to reckon with psychotropic drugs as a major reason for these increases. For example, the state of Georgia's costs for psychotropics used in prisons increased from $4,498,109 in fiscal year 2000

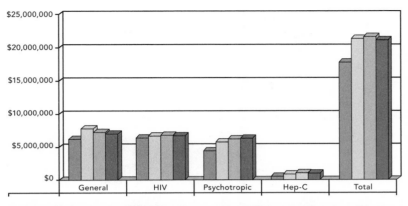

	General	HIV	Psycho-tropics	Hepatitis C	Total
FY 2000	$6,227,187	$6,507,098	$4,498,109	$617,145	$17,849,539
FY 2001	$7,853,752	$6,833,723	$5,811,085	$898,328	$21,396,888
FY 2002	$7,313,218	$6,892,294	$6,254,827	$1,138,139	$21,598,478
FY 2003	$7,057,485	$6,807,046	$6,377,498	$1,052,937	$21,254,957

FIGURE 3. Drug expenditures in Georgia prisons, FY 2000–FY 2003.

to $6,337,498 in fiscal year 2003, as shown in Figure 3. The outsourcing of prisoner health care services to for-profit corporations represents one popular strategy to reduce costs. However, in terms of cost savings, prison health care privatization has been a failure. A 2011 report on prison health care in Pennsylvania notes that "the history of contracted prison healthcare both in Pennsylvania and across the country is a history of unrealized cost savings, lawsuits, and diminished care."[17] A 2001 U.S. Bureau of Justice Assistance study on prison privatization found that private prisons offered only 1 percent cost savings on average, and the savings were achieved primarily through lower labor costs.[18]

(MIS)MANAGING THE INVENTORY

One strategy some prisons have used to try to contain costs has been to procure pharmacy inventory management technology. Controlling inventory is a major problem for prison pharmacies, where inadequate inventory systems can increase the likelihood of worker fraud, abuse, and theft. The strategy of putting new inventory technologies in place has exposed an especially troubling dysfunction when it comes to basic pharmacy record keeping.

Consider the case of Iowa. The state is ranked nearly last in the nation in prison spending (forty-ninth) and near the bottom in imprisonment rates (fortieth). Nearly half of its prisoners have been diagnosed with mental illness (46.2 percent), and 29.5 percent of that group have serious mental disorders, such as chronic schizophrenia, recurrent major depressive disorder, bipolar disorder, other chronic and recurrent psychosis, and organic neurological disorders. On August 1, 2000, Iowa's state prison system began using a new networked software platform, Iowa Correction Offender Network, or ICON, to manage a wide range of information about prisoners, including data from clinical, psychological, and criminological assessments.[19] ICON replaced two older mainframe systems—ACIS and ICDC—that provided browser functionality and remote access to information.[20] According to the Iowa audit report, ICON is supposed to improve the standards of mental health care "by using 'wizards' to direct users to consistently collect all necessary information needed to make more informed assessments and diagnoses."[21] Figure 4 is a screenshot of the ICON system at work. The offender, oddly represented by a personal computer in the center of the image, is surrounded by concentric circles of generalized "processes" that link the offender to service providers (medical, dental, laboratory, mental health, and optometry) within an overarching service management structure that features physician orders; automatic, one-time, and recurrent inmate appointment scheduling; and workload forecasting and management.

Now, let's turn to Colorado, where in 2005 prison pharmacies filled over 262,200 inmate prescriptions, more than 700 per day on average. The most common prescriptions were for "cardiovascular, psychotropic, nonsteroidal anti-inflammatory, and gastrointestinal medications."[22] The Department of Corrections spent $8.4 million on medications in 2005. Auditors later found that the department's inventory data were neither accurate nor reliable. No controls were in place to ensure that staff followed through and transferred manually recorded prescription data into the electronic system. Drug destruction was also an issue. Medications were not supposed to be destroyed at clinics, yet staff at six clinics destroyed medicines on-site when inmates refused them. The auditors wrote: "No record of the exact number of pills destroyed exists. Further, the clinics employ various methods for destroying medications. For ex-

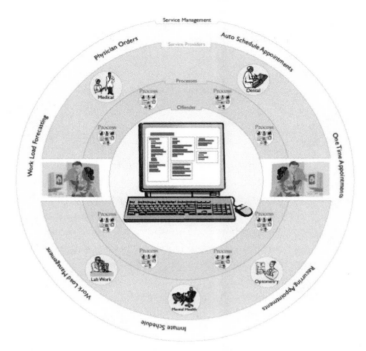

FIGURE 4. Iowa Correction Offender Network (ICON) at work.

ample, one facility crushes the medication and pours it down the sink drain. Another facility places the medication in a trash receptacle that is handled by an inmate porter. In both cases, no witness is required when the medication is disposed of or destroyed."[23] In regard to these practices, the auditors noted, "We consider this issue a critical one because the risk for fraud and abuse is high."[24]

In 2007–8, the North Carolina Division of Prisons Central Pharmacy spent about $25.1 million for drugs and pharmaceutical supplies for the prison population. Although it dispensed more than 4,800 medications daily, the auditors found,

> the Central Pharmacy does not maintain adequate control over inventory access to prevent unauthorized use, theft, or loss of approximately $25.1 million in drug and pharmaceutical supply purchases. Nor does it maintain adequate records to ensure that recorded inventory balances are accurate. The results of two separate inventory counts, one performed by Central Pharmacy

staff and one performed by auditors, provide evidence that Central Pharmacy physical access and record-keeping controls are inadequate. Additionally, pharmacists were observed removing items from the Central Pharmacy stockroom without requesting items from stockroom staff, and Central Pharmacy employees with access to pharmacy inventory also had the ability to adjust inventory records. Inadequate inventory controls expose the Central Pharmacy inventory to the risk of unauthorized use, theft, and loss.[25]

The North Carolina situation is similar to that in King County, Washington, where audits of pharmacy operations were initiated in response to an ombudsman report citing inmate complaints regarding timeliness and accuracy of prescriptions, concerns about workload among staff of the jail health services, reliance on temporary agency nurses, ineffective improvement programs, and deficiencies noted in a State Board of Pharmacy inspection report. Auditors found a theme within the jail— that its mission was "to secure custody" rather than "to provide health services."[26] Under the existing system, medications were often lost or went missing. The auditors specified four types of incidents that accounted for problems with the inventory record: *miscellaneous incidents,* which included count discrepancies, unsecured prescriptions, and use of expired medications; *dispensing incidents,* which involved incorrect medications or doses provided to inmates, medications dispensed but not administered, and medications dispensed without orders; *transcription incidents,* which involved duplicate or missing orders; and *ordering incidents,* those in which orders were confusing, incorrect, or incomplete.[27]

Vermont first tried using for-profit correctional health care providers in 1996, a move that the state hoped would help with inventory problems. A 2013 audit there illuminated specific conflicts over data from the private health care contractor, Correct Care Solutions (CCS). The problem was that "CCS did not always provide required operational reports or the reports did not contain all required information. . . . For example, in December 2010, DOC sent CCS a summary of the first year of the contract in which it stated that 'there are a number of inaccuracies in both CCS financial and statistical reports and this is not acceptable. Data parameters that were agreed upon . . . have not been reported.'"[28] In fact, the auditors noted, the DOC health services director had complained, "It seems that the whole notion of creating reports for the purpose of documenting care and services and assessing performance were [sic] not taken seriously by CCS. There was no expectation that they would be paying penalties."[29] The monitoring and quality assurance data that CCS was supposed to give the Vermont Department of Corrections were at least eighteen months overdue, and the "animosity surrounding the report requirements and objections by CCS over penalties were beginning to taint negotiations for a contract extension, which were occurring at the same time."[30]

CONTROLLING PSYCHOTROPIC DRUG COSTS

Shifting from expensive patent-protected psychotropics to cheaper but no less effective generic medications has been another approach to lowering costs. New Hampshire was looking for cost savings due to the high costs of "recidivism, the loss of Medicaid for inmates while in prison, expensive psychotropic drugs, an expensive contract with Dartmouth Medical School (DMS), and a growing elderly population in prisons."[31] The auditors noted that in FY 2006, the state's Division of Medical and Forensic Services, which was "responsible for coordinating the physical and mental health of all inmates spent a total of $8,275,000, or 9.2 percent of the total Corrections budget."[32] Of that amount, $1,058,600 was spent to dispense 19,030 prescriptions for psychotropic medications. These figures were up from FY 2004 ($698,300 for 16,399 prescriptions) and FY 2005 ($861,700 for 18,105 prescriptions). The auditors found that

> at any given point in time, 25 to 35 percent of state inmates use psychotropic medications, and the number of these medications has increased over the past few years. . . . This increase may be partially correlated with the growing elderly population in the correctional system and the subsequent increase in demand for psychotropic medications. In addition, the cost of psychotropic medications has increased nationally. The state uses expensive brand name medications, such as the anti-psychotic medication Seroquel, as opposed to less expensive generic medications.[33]

Among the policy options the auditors proposed to help reduce the costs of mental health care for inmates were the following: creation of diversion programs based on models from other jurisdictions, continuation and broadening of the use of mental health courts, the use of telemedicine, and a switch to the use of generic psychotropic medications.[34]

To reduce the costs of psychotropic medications, the auditors advised, New Hampshire should look to the examples of other states, like Vermont, which "cut down Seroquel's use from 110 prescriptions in 2006 to five prescriptions in 2007."[35]

Psychotropic drugs accounted for more than half (58 percent) of all medication costs at Utah's Salt Lake County Adult Detention Center during the audit period of December 2000 through May 2006. Accumulatively, there were 53,138 inmates on medications, 40.77 percent of whom (21,662) were on psychotropics, which cost the county more than $2.48 million. The auditors focused on psychotropics because approximately half of inmates who were being prescribed any medication type were receiving psychotropics. More than half of all medication costs were for SSRIs and atypical antipsychotic medications. These two kinds of drugs were considered more effective than other psychotropics at reducing symptoms and improving cognitive function, and they produced fewer side effects, although in this case *fewer* often just means *different* side effects.

The Salt Lake County auditors found that expenditures on medications had increased 550 percent over the prior ten years: from $146,374 in 1996 to $957,355 in 2005 (49,041 prescriptions). In 2004, a 36 percent increase in the detention center's drug costs (from $785,601 to $1,071,824) was attributed, in part, to increased use of psychotropic medications for treatment of depression and mental illness.[36] In that year, the facility signed a contract with a new for-profit provider of mental health services, which "relied on the use of expensive psychotropic medications in the absence of qualified staff to pursue less costly educational counseling and therapeutic alternatives."[37] In addition, the auditors cited as reasons for the 2004 increase the lack of a formulary guide, lack of qualified staff, and the fact that discount coupons for certain medications, such as Zyprexa, were no longer available. For example, a coupon for Zyprexa that phased out in 2004 had accounted for a savings of $20,000 per month during 2002 and 2003. Staffing mental health managers was also problematic—within a period of eighteen months, three were hired and then either were fired or resigned.

The auditors also determined that procedures for tracking pills were insufficient to ensure that drugs were not stolen. In fact, during the audit period, a pharmacy technician stole ninety Lortab pills. In discussing this event, the auditors wrote, "While Jail medical staff does track individual pills within each bottle or on each blister pack, and in fact, double counts these pills twice a day, no overall inventory control sheet is used to list each bottle or blister pack in the controlled substance cabinet."[38]

In Salt Lake County, prescriptions for psychotropics are written by psychiatrists, advanced practice registered nurses, general medical doctors, physicians' assistants, and nurse practitioners. In addition to presenting their findings, the auditors made this telling observation: "An on-going policy debate exists regarding the role correctional institutions should play in the treatment and care of the mentally ill. An individual's mental state may contribute to criminal or offensive behavior. Some 'crimes' committed by the mentally ill are misdemeanors, such as indecent exposure or other unusual behavior, but may result in incarceration to remove a nuisance or potential threat from public view. For many mentally ill individuals jail is a revolving door of incarceration and repeated bookings that can and do occur repeatedly over time."[39]

Auditors in Allegany County, New York, found that 2,100 prescriptions for inmates had been filled at a local pharmacy in 2012, at a total cost of more than $198,000. The auditors noted that "county officials did not retain documentation to indicate how [drug] prices were determined and do not verify that the prices being charged are in keeping with the verbal agreement" the county had with the pharmacy to charge a lower rate than the national price list.[40] The county officials argued that using the local, and probably more expensive, pharmacy was preferable for reasons other than cost. They noted that a prison pharmacy can be a local economic enterprise, providing jobs and cash to local businesses. In their response to the auditors' comments, the county officials wrote:

> The pharmacy being used sits down the hill from the County Courthouse and old County Jail and a little over a mile north of the current Jail. The pharmacy has been providing prescription medications to the Jail for more than 20 years. It is owned and operated by a local pharmacist and provides not only excellent and critical services, but the owner and employees of this business own homes and invest money in the local community. . . .
>
> . . . Yes, the County may be able to buy drugs cheaper somewhere else, but that is not the only cost involved. We are involved in securing a professional service and not a mere commodity. If a true emergency were to arise and we needed those services outside

normal business hours, we are confident they will be provided. Having confidence in a professional is not something that can easily be quantified. . . . We respectfully disagree with some of the conclusions relative to the value of the services provided.[41]

The state of Wisconsin has conducted two audits of its prison health care systems, one in 2001 focused on prison health care in general and the other in 2009 focused on prison mental health care. The first audit was conducted in response to the death of inmate Michelle Grier from an asthma attack; she was twenty-nine years old when she died on February 2, 2000, an event that "raised concerns about inmates' access to health services and the quality of those services."[42] That day, Grier told guards that her rescue inhaler was not working and asked to go the medical clinic; she was seen by a nurse, who told Grier that because she "was walking and could be understood, she was not having an asthma attack."[43] Grier collapsed a short time later, having suffered cardiac arrest as a result of the attack. Stories like this rarely see the light of day.

The Wisconsin Department of Corrections operates medical clinics in its fourteen adult facilities, which served approximately 14,900 prisoners in FY 1999–2000. Additional care was provided at the University of Wisconsin hospitals, at local hospitals, in a sixty-four-bed infirmary at the Dodge Correctional Institution, and in specialized psychological services units in three prisons and two other public mental health institutions. Prison health care expenditures increased dramatically in Wisconsin from FY 1994–95 to FY 1999–2000, out of proportion to the modest increases in the prison population. Expenditures for pharmaceuticals alone increased 400 percent during this period. The system spent $6.6 million on pharmaceuticals in FY 1999–2000, with five psychotropics among the top six drug expenditures: Seroquel and Risperdal (antipsychotics), Paxil and Zoloft (depression), and Neurontin (mood stabilizer). Eleven of the top twenty drug expenditures were for psychotropics.[44] The number of psychiatric prescription orders rose by 68 percent from FY 1996–97 to FY 1999–2000.[45] Yet, the auditors who conducted Wisconsin's 2009 audit noted that in 2001 the Department of Corrections (DOC) did not maintain statistics on the numbers of inmates with diagnosed mental illnesses.[46] Estimates of the number of inmates with mental illnesses were based on prescriptions provided by the DOC and on the number who were receiving treatment from DOC psychiatrists. The auditors observed: "This estimate likely undercounted the number of mentally ill inmates, and the lack of a consistent classification system made it difficult for DOC or others to assess mental health care needs in state prisons."[47] Prescriptions for inmates are filled by the Bureau of Health Services Central Pharmacy, which buys drugs in bulk through MMCAP (described above). Emergency prescriptions are filled locally.

The 2009 Wisconsin audit found that mental health care costs continued to increase, from $46.1 million in FY 2003–4 to $59.8 million in FY 2007–8.[48] The cost of psychotropic medications ranged from $4.6 million to a high of $6.1 million in FY 2007–8. But, the auditors found, "the number of psychotropic medication orders [the Central Pharmacy] filled increased by 32.6 percent from FY 2003–04 through FY 2007–08, while expenditures for psychotropic medications increased by only 13.0 percent. The difference suggests that DOC's efforts to limit costs have been successful."[49] Antidepressants are the most commonly prescribed psychotropic medications, and two of the top ten psychotropics are antipsychotics. At about two-thirds of psychiatry appointments, medications are adjusted (rather than discontinued). While the DOC aimed to prescribe medications from the formulary, 96.8 percent of all requests for nonformulary psychotropic medications were approved.[50] Figure 5 lists the psychotropics most commonly prescribed as found in the 2009 Wisconsin audit.

In mid-2004, the Wisconsin DOC began to score inmates' mental health along a continuum ranging from no mental health needs to serious mental health needs.[51] There is no standardization of mental health scoring across jurisdictions, however. Inmates are classified according to the severity of their illness: the classification MH-0 indicates no mental illness, MH-1 is for inmates who have some mental health needs but are not seriously mentally ill, and MH-2 is for inmates who are seriously mentally ill. MH-1 includes inmates with short-term diagnoses, who do not meet criteria for formal diagnoses, or whose illnesses are not as extreme as those of prisoners classified as MH-2. An inmate is considered to be mentally ill if he or she fits the requirements for classification as MH-1 or MH-2. There is no automation of diagnoses, and some inmates are diagnosed for multiple illnesses; the classifications are not consistently documented or routinely updated.[52]

While prisons have developed processes for classifying inmates so that they can receive mental health care, these processes are not always

Drug Name (Brand)	Commonly Prescribed for	Number of Inmates with Prescriptions
Trazodone (Desyrel)	Depression	694
Fluoxetine (Prozac)	Depression	686
Citalopram (Celexa)	Depression	627
Mirtazapine (Remeron)	Depression	462
Diphenhydramine (Benadryl)	Allergies, sleep disorders	441
Risperidone (Risperdal)	Psychotic disorders	402
Amitriptyline (Elavil)	Depression	333
Quetiapine (Seroquel)	Psychotic disorders	333
Hydroxyzine (Atarax, Vistaril)	Anxiety	275
Venlafaxine (Effexor)	Depression	259
Bupropion (Wellbutrin)	Depression	249
Lithium (Eskalith, Lithobid)	Bipolar disorder	244
Valproic acid (Depakene)	Seizure disorders, bipolar disorder	219
Ziprasidone (Geodon)	Psychotic disorders	213
Benzatropine (Cogentin)	Side effects associated with antipsychotic medications	201
Clonazepam (Klonopin)	Panic disorders	172
Buspirone (Buspar)	Anxiety	171
Sertraline (Zoloft)	Depression, anxiety	166
Paroxetine (Paxil)	Depression, anxiety	142
Doxepin (Sinequan)	Depression, anxiety	105

FIGURE 5. Most commonly prescribed psychotropics according to the 2009 Wisconsin audit. Brand names are listed for reference; the Wisconsin Department of Corrections reports using generic medications when available. Some drugs may be prescribed for uses other than those listed, and inmates may be prescribed more than one psychotropic medication.

followed. In Wisconsin, any inmate who is prescribed a psychotropic is supposed to be classified as MH-1 or MH-2. The Wisconsin auditors discovered, however, that for a two-year period, 190 inmates were prescribed psychotropic medications even though they were not coded as having mental health needs.[53] The auditors noted that while "reliable and comparable data are not readily available on a national basis, research suggests that the gender and racial/ethnic differences among DOC inmates are consistent with national trends. DOC officials attribute these differences, in part, to gender and cultural differences in inmates' willingness to seek mental health care."[54] Without proper psychiatric assessments and consistent documentation of those assessments, it is difficult to determine whether prescribing practices are sound and reasonable. Without any analysis of how differences in drug treatment among gender, racial, and age groups might result from institutional policies, Wisconsin is left to rely on problematic assumptions rather than on reliable data.

In terms of drug delivery, most medications are administered by correctional officers rather than by psychiatrists, nurses, or other health care staff. Yet correctional officers are typically not informed of inmates' mental health status, nor are they trained to identify side effects of medications. "For example," the 2001 Wisconsin auditors explained, "some psychotropic medications can have serious withdrawal symptoms if stopped abruptly. Staff reported several instances of inmates experiencing severe withdrawal symptoms when medications were interrupted because of problems with correctional officers getting medications to inmates."[55]

A 2011 Michigan audit report noted that "the number of prisoners receiving mental health outpatient treatment and psychotropic medications has more than doubled from 2,000 in 2004–2005 to over 5,000 in 2010. Because psychotropic medications are restricted and require individual distribution by health care staff, this has significantly increased health care staff work load."[56] Interestingly, the prisoner count in Michigan was declining at that time, but pharmaceutical costs were rising. Figure 6 compares the state's average prisoner count to its total prison pharmaceutical costs. The auditors found that the DOC's efforts "to manage prisoner pharmaceutical costs were not effective."[57] Insufficient procedures and inadequate contract language, insufficient refill process controls, and approval of nonformulary prescriptions also fueled costs.

From January 1 to July 31, 2010, the Michigan DOC spent $8,473,320 on psychotropic drugs, an expenditure that represented 41 percent of pharmaceutical expenditures for that period. The other drug categories noted by the auditors were general medicine (29 percent at $6,153,198), HIV (16 percent at $3,262,096), gastrointestinal (7 percent at $1,529,604),

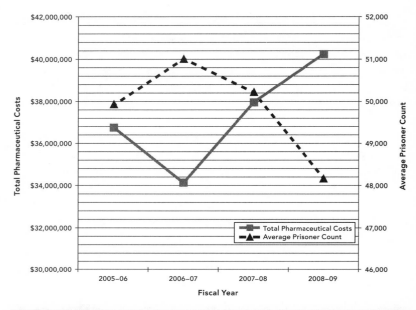

Fiscal Year	Total Pharmaceutical Costs	Average Prisoner Count	Average Pharmaceutical Cost per Prisoner
2005–6	$36,751,745	49,916	$736
2006–7	$34,123,648	51,020	$669
2007–8	$37,961,069	50,232	$756
2008–9	$40,231,125	48,170	$835

FIGURE 6. Prison pharmaceutical costs in Michigan: comparison of total pharmaceutical costs and average prisoner count, FY 2005–6 through FY 2008–9. The Michigan Office of the Auditor General prepared this exhibit based on unaudited accounting records and prisoner census reports obtained from the Department of Corrections.

and cardiovascular (7 percent at $1,455,390).[58] Figure 7 gives a detailed breakdown of the costs for drugs in the psychotropic category.

Prior to the audit, Michigan had not implemented any measures to contain the high costs represented by the prescription of atypical antipsychotics such as Abilify, Geodon, Invega, Risperdal, Seroquel, and Zyprexa. In a letter to the Department of Corrections in June 2009, the former medical services contractor reported that Seroquel prescriptions "were nine times the average of other states for which the

Drug, Category	Total Cost	Percentage of Total Cost
Seroquel, atypical antipsychotic	$4,526,473	62 percent
Zyprexa, atypical antipsychotic	$1,022,106	14 percent
Abilify, atypical antipsychotic	$1,101,531	13 percent
Second-generation antidepressants	$454,268	5 percent
Mood stabilizers	$279,828	3 percent
Typical antipsychotics	$206,120	2 percent
Other psychotics	$140,136	1 percent
First-generation antidepressants	$67,212	less than 1 percent
Sedative/hypnotics	$24,992	less than 1 percent

FIGURE 7. Breakdown of costs of psychotropics in the Michigan Department of Corrections.

contractor provided statewide prison pharmaceutical services and in which Seroquel was targeted for reduction."[59] Risperdal is an "industry recognized lower-cost alternative to Seroquel," which was still on patent. The auditors noted that factors other than cost (such as medical, safety, and security concerns) would have to be evaluated before Risperdal could be substituted for Seroquel, but they believed it would be cost-beneficial to evaluate such options for the most prescribed and most costly atypical antipsychotic medications. They produced the data shown in Figure 8 to enumerate the potential savings of shifting from Seroquel to Risperdal.

The auditors found that the DOC's efforts to control and safeguard prisoner pharmaceuticals had not been effective in the areas of receiving, maintaining, and distributing prisoner "medications such as Atripla, Catapres, Norvir, Truvada, Ultram, Zyprexa, and other psychiatric drugs that can be expensive and have a high potential for abuse. At 9 of the 10 locations, health care staff did not document or ensure that there was a witness to the disposal of medications. . . . The lack of controls over the disposal process may facilitate and conceal loss or theft of medications. We observed varying amounts of individual pills discarded in sharps containers. . . . [Some containers] appeared to contain thousands of discarded pills."[60] The DOC's response to the audit was to create a consolidated mental health system that would be under the direction of the DOC chief psychiatric officer. During the first 180 days of the

Percentage reduction in Seroquel	10 percent	25 percent	33 percent	50 percent	75 percent	100 percent
Average monthly number of Seroquel prescriptions	2,386	2,386	2,386	2,386	2,386	2,386
Potential reduction in number of Seroquel prescriptions	239	597	787	1,193	1,790	2,386
Average monthly cost of Seroquel prescription	$335	$335	$335	$335	$335	$335
Projected reduction in Seroquel cost	$80,065	$119,995	$263,645	$339,665	$559,650	$799,310
Average monthly cost of Risperdal prescription	$38	$38	$38	$38	$38	$38
Projected increase in Risperdal cost	$9,082	$22,686	$29,906	$45,334	$68,020	$90,668
Average monthly reduction in cost	$70,983	$117,309	$233,739	$354,321	$531,630	$708,642
Annualized potential savings	$851,796	$2,127,708	$2,804,868	$4,251,852	$6,379,560	$8,503,704

FIGURE 8. Potential savings of switching antipsychotics: from Seroquel to Risperdal.

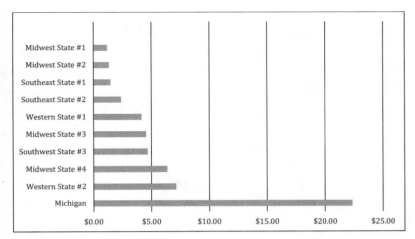

FIGURE 9. Michigan audit, comparisons of antipsychotic costs, 2010. For these ten states, the Department of Corrections contracts with PharmaCorr for statewide pharmacy services. About 80 percent of Michigan's atypical antipsychotic medications prescribed for DOC prisoners are written by the Department of Community Health and contracted psychiatrists. Source: DOC's pharmacy contractor.

consolidation, "all existing atypical antipsychotic prisoner prescription medications will be reviewed through a new process which includes the addition of a utilization management nurse to strengthen provider education about efficacy, cost, and alternatives during the process."[61] As Figure 9 from the audit shows, Michigan's antipsychotic expenditures were completely out of sync with those of other states.

THE PROBLEM OF WASTE

California prison pharmacies provide good examples of how wasteful prison pharmacies can be. In 2010, the state of California's Office of the Inspector General conducted an audit of prison pharmacies in response to concerns expressed by pharmacy staff during regular inspections about "the sheer amount of wasted medication in prison pharmacies."[62] Back in October 2005, the U.S. Northern District Court had forced the California Department of Corrections and Rehabilitation (CDCR) into receivership because of its failure to provide constitutionally adequate medical care to prisoners. "The court found CDCR prison pharmacy operations, in particular, to be 'unbelievably poor.'"[63] The receiver contracted with Maxor National Pharmacy Services to assist in and help improve CDCR's pharmacy operations. As the auditors related,

"In June 2006, Maxor concluded its review and issued a report titled, 'An Analysis of the Crisis in the California Prison Pharmacy System Including a Road Map from Despair to Excellence.' In this report, Maxor asserted that the 'CDCR pharmacy program does not meet minimal standards of patient care, provide inventory controls or ensure standardization.'"[64]

From 2000 to 2008, the amount of money the CDCR spent on medications doubled, while the prison population increased only 7 percent and drug costs increased only 33 percent.[65] Unfortunately, as the auditors found, this trend continued through 2010. They noted that, "contrary to expectation, there are almost no procedures for identifying and restocking medications." Pharmacists were trying to "find ways around the state-wide computerized inventory system, a system so unreliable that pharmacists prefer to rely on handwritten tallies."[66] The auditors' general findings were as follows:

> Usable medications not being restocked in prison pharmacies [and instead being disposed of] cost California taxpayers at least $7.7 million annually.
>
> Not ensuring the use of approved medications costs California taxpayers an additional $5.5 million annually.
>
> Unreliable computer inventories in prison pharmacies result in additional staff labor and increased costs.
>
> Inconsistent practices in handling medications for inmates who transfer between prisons result in waste and increased costs.[67]

The auditors reported that they "observed large quantities of returned medications stored in tote bins and plastic bags, waiting to be sorted."[68]

They stated further: "In its 2006 review of CDCR pharmacies, Maxor noted significant inventory problems, noting that 'based on a sampling of selected medications, it appears that millions of dollars of purchased medications are not accounted for in the prescription dispensing data.' In the same report, Maxor observed, 'Such disturbing variances (in excess of 30%) indicate a serious lack of pharmacy management and inventory control, as well as a high level of waste and potential for drug diversion.'"[69]

Maxor's solution to the problem was to install a computerized inventory system—GuardianRx—which had been in use for six months at the time of the 2010 audit. "However," the auditors reported, "most pharmacy staff told inspectors that the new computer inventory system

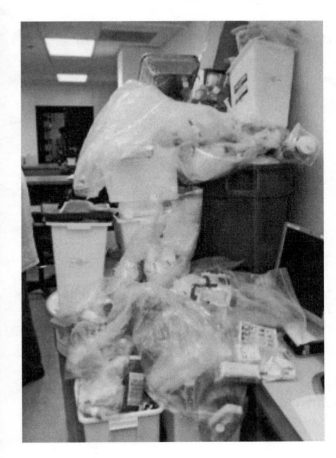

FIGURE 10.
Returned
unused
medication
in California.

was not accurate and could not be trusted. While visiting one pharmacy, an inspector took a bottle of medication from a shelf and asked the pharmacist if anyone would notice if he removed the bottle. The pharmacist replied, 'Probably not.' Pharmacy staff at three additional institutions gave similar answers."[70] The auditors selected fourteen medications from the most expensive ones stocked in prison pharmacies and compared the physical inventory with the computer inventory for each drug. "The most significant disparity was in Risperidone 3mg., of which inspectors counted 5,191 actual tablets while the computer inventory indicated a stock of 24,360 tablets. This is a difference of 470 percent. The discrepancy between the computer inventory and the physical inventory of these medications demonstrates the unreliability of this system."[71] The auditors also found that the practices for handling medications for inmates who transferred between prisons were inconsistent, resulting in waste and increased costs. "We discovered that once inmates arrive at the receiving prison, all of their medications are refilled, regardless of the amount of medication sent from the previous prison. All extra medications are returned to the receiving prison pharmacy, where it is highly unlikely they are restocked."[72]

At the federal level, things are not much different. The mission of the Federal Bureau of Prison (BOP) Pharmacy Services, a part of the broader BOP Health Services Division, is to "provide access for inmates to quality, necessary, and cost-effective drug care consistent with community standards."[73] The "cost-effective" part of this mission was under assault in the early 2000s, as health care expenditures increased from $412.65 million in FY 2000 to $623.52 million in FY 2004. Prescription medication costs also increased over this period, rising from 5.5 percent of total health care costs in FY 2000 to 8.1 percent in FY 2004. Hence the need for an audit by the Department of Justice's Office of the Inspector General to evaluate the BOP's efforts to reduce costs, assess controls and safeguards over medications, and ensure compliance with laws and policies.[74] Overall, the auditors concluded that

> the BOP has not adequately assessed the budgetary impact of its initiatives to reduce increasing costs for prescription medications. . . . We also found that the BOP's cost-benefit analysis for its Central Fill proposal contained errors and incorrect assumptions that may result in increased prescription medication costs rather than savings. We also found that the BOP needs to improve efforts to reduce prescription medication costs associated with waste and ensure that cost savings initiatives such as the OTC policy are fully implemented.[75]

Unlike the state prison systems, the BOP uses the Federal Supply Schedule to guide its prescription medication purchases. As the auditors described it, "The FSS is a price catalog of over 23,000 prescription medications that are available for purchase by federal agencies. In addition to the FSS, the BOP utilizes specific contracts with prescription medication companies administered by the Veterans Administration (VA). The BOP purchases over 40 prescription medications through 'Mandatory National Contracts' administered by the VA, which require that each institution buy specific medication brands."[76]

In fiscal year 2004, psychotropics accounted for 23 percent of the BOP's total prescription costs, about $12 million.[77] The auditors found that 6,910 inmates were being treated with one or more psychotropic drugs as of March 2005, although in a footnote they pointed out that, because of differences in drug tracking practices, this number did not include information from the Oklahoma Federal Transfer Center, the Rochester Medical Center, or the Beaumont Federal Correctional Complex.[78] The federal inspectors identified a series of problems, including a lack of adequate controls over purchasing, the filling of prescriptions that had not been signed by doctors or pharmacists, missing information in inmate medical files, and a range of concerns about controlled substances.[79] The lack of controls allowed the chief pharmacist at the El Reno Federal Correctional Institution to steal 30,600 doses of prescription medications for his personal use between July 2002 and February 2004.[80]

The only prison pharmacy audit that seriously raised the question of the possible misuse of psychotropics was a 2014 audit of health services in the Minnesota Department of Corrections. DOC medical staff told the auditors that "offenders were receiving too many prescriptions for psychotropic drugs, narcotics, sedatives, and a pain reliever called gabapentin (or Neurontin)."[81] The auditors examined some unspecified "system-wide trends in the number of orders for these medications from the first six months of 2010 to the first six months of 2013" and found that costs for these drugs went down, and that prescriptions for these drugs were also down, but only marginally.[82] But costs for Neurontin in the St. Cloud Prison *increased 94 percent,* and costs for psychotropics in the Moose Lake/Willow River Facility *increased 107 percent* over this period. "Thus," the auditors concluded, "there may be differences in the prescription patterns of individual practitioners that require additional attention. But," they added, "in general, the concerns we heard about escalating use and cost of prescription pharmaceuticals were not borne out by our review of system-wide data."[83]

The auditors then proceeded to sidestep this central medical, ethical, and legal question raised by prison medical staff. Their response was typical of these prison pharmacy audits generally:

We offer no judgments about the appropriateness of prescription practices from a clinical perspective. Some medical staff expressed concern to us that the prisons rely too much on medications and not enough on patient education, or that the formulary medications are less effective or have more adverse side effects than alternatives that are not on the formulary. There may be valid concerns about the merits of particular medications prescribed to offenders, but we did not have the expertise to explore them.[84]

Well, then, nothing to see here. Case closed.

Through these prison pharmacy audits, we see the scope and dynamics of prescription drug distribution and learn about the management problems that define this critical part of prison health care. In short, prison pharmacies are a management nightmare, and their dysfunction should raise concerns about the standards of health care practiced in confinement settings and the mechanisms of accountability linked to those standards. It does not seem like an exaggeration to suggest that no one is monitoring the prison pharmacy counter.

THREE

EXPERIMENTAL PATRIOTS

Citizenship and the Racial Ethics of Prison Drug Testing

In chapters 1 and 2, we have explored some of what we know and do not know about the use of psychotropics in U.S. prisons. Together, these two chapters paint a picture of vast amounts of government-produced ignorance, medical incompetence, and bureaucratic malfeasance surrounding psychotropics and their role in mass captivity. From the prisoner health surveys and institutional censuses, we can construct only a partial understanding of how psychotropics are distributed within prisons, an understanding that suggests that government officials have not been particularly interested in knowing more about drugging practices. If they were more interested, perhaps they would have paid closer attention to the questions that have been asked of prison authorities and prisoners over decades of research. When we look at the audits of contemporary prison pharmacies, the one place from which we might extract a fuller accounting of psychotropic distribution, we see institutions that have a bureaucratic fixation on lowering costs. Prison pharmacies are struggling to manage the flow of all drugs, not just psychotropics, through the prisons and into prisoners' minds and bodies.

Because state and federal governments did not begin to collect and publish data about drug distribution in prisons until the mid-1970s, both of the preceding chapters have focused on relatively recent history, concentrating mainly on what we can and cannot know in the contemporary period. If what we can know about how psychotropics are used *now* is constrained by institutional factors, what can we know about how psychotropics were used *before* the mid-1970s? If we have only partial information about how psychotropics circulate in the prisons now, can we determine when psychotropics first entered the prisons? How did they get inside in the first place? The simple answer to this question is that the U.S. pharmaceutical industry has been situated in prisons all over the country for nearly one hundred years, having set up shop there in the 1920s and 1930s. When psychotropics were first manufactured in the 1950s, prisons were already fertile ground for the biomedical experimentation required for these drugs' mass production and distribution. The more complicated answer to this question is the subject of this chapter. To interrogate the issue of how psychotropics entered the prisons, I analyze documents submitted to the National Commission for the Protection of Human Subjects of Biomedical and Behavioral Research, which was active from 1974 to 1978.[1] A rhetoric of citizenship framed how drug companies positioned prisoners' participation in drug tests, with the companies depicting such participation as an altruistic act of patriotism and an exercise of citizenship. This rhetoric was shaped by the racial biopolitics of participation in prison drug studies that was dominant at the time.

No one knows precisely how many imprisoned citizens have been subjected against their will or without their knowledge to patch tests, no-name pills, malaria-infected mosquitoes, countless blood draws, or irradiation of the testicles since the first drug studies were conducted on U.S. prisoners in the late 1920s. No comprehensive public accounting of prison drug studies has ever been compiled by researchers, government officials, or drug companies. Even the most careful historians of human experimentation in prisons have been forced to string together a hodgepodge of cases, those rare instances where the documentary record provides enough information that making reasonable claims about the practice is warranted.[2] To my knowledge, no scholars have yet focused on clinical trials in their efforts to document the extent of human experimentation in prisons.

The pharmaceutical industry has been and remains a powerful institutional force inside U.S. prisons, having developed extensive drug testing programs throughout federal and state prison systems. The use of U.S. prisoners as research subjects in drug tests accelerated during World War II and the postwar period.[3] Then, between 1962 and the mid-1970s, "virtually all" of the human research subjects used in safety and bioavailability studies of new drug compounds were prisoners.[4] According to the National Commission for the Protection of Human Subjects of Biomedical and Behavioral Research, in 1975, fourteen drug companies were conducting one hundred different studies of seventy-one individual compounds on about 3,600 prisoners.[5] That was just one year's worth of experimentation.

Decades of largely unfettered access to prisons as sampling grounds for new drug experiments (presumably) helped to lower pharmaceutical companies' costs of developing new drugs, which in turn increased their profits. Undoubtedly, the availability of prisoners helped to position the pharmaceutical industry as one of the most profitable sectors in contemporary global capitalism. For years, prisoners represented a site for the primitive accumulation of biocapital that would generate billions for drug companies and scientific esteem for hundreds of research scientists.[6] The proposition that prison drug experimentation was ethical provided convenient cover for the long-standing financial and political relationships between U.S. drug companies and prisons. This special partnership, quite lucrative for the drug firms and politically useful for prisons, began with drug companies and researchers convincing prison officials that male prisoners represented ideal research subjects for pharmaceutical products because of the prisons' central locations and the open work schedules, standardized diets, and regimented daily activities of the inmates.

We might be tempted to believe that, given the racial segregation that defines the U.S. prison system, the drug testing programs targeted black bodies for data extraction and capitalist exploitation. This was my assumption when I started poking around this history. But scholars working at the intersection of black studies, technology, and medicine, motivated by a desire to document how black bodies have been targeted and exploited by medical science, face a daunting investigational challenge in the context of prisons.[7] The archival records of prison drug testing that historians have unearthed barely breathe a word about black prisoners' participation in these studies. In her book *Medical Apartheid*, perhaps the most exhaustive accounting of medical experimentation on black people to date, Harriet Washington stitches together a series of experiments that feature black prisoners as research subjects.[8] Basing her discussion heavily on Allen Hornblum's research in *Acres of Skin*, Washington presents the racial history of prison experimentation as one that explicitly targets black prisoners, often drawing on theories of black degeneracy and inferiority.[9] From 1962 to 1979, the most active years of the prison drug testing programs, researchers were focused on carrying out drug trials on whatever bodies they could for as cheaply as they could—they did not seem particularly interested in recruiting black people. Given the lack of available information, however, it is impossible to discern precisely how race shaped drug companies' sampling procedures in their prison-based drug trials. We do not know how drug testing programs were connected to racial hierarchies, and there is near radio silence on the participation of black prisoners in studies of psychotropic drugs, a consequence of the secrecy attached to prison experimentation.

Participation in prison drug testing was linked to citizenship in ways that validated white prisoners' sense of patriotism. By volunteering to be subjects in drug studies, white male prisoners could demonstrate that they were moral actors and good citizens. These "experimental patriots" also embodied a discourse that aimed to justify the ongoing use of prisoners as subjects in drug studies. The national imperative to develop pharmaceutical agents that could be used to treat diseases of war (e.g., malaria) or be used as weapons of war became paramount in the already robust business of drug testing in U.S. prisons. Nazi doctors had made similar "conditions of war" justifications for some of their inhumane medical experiments conducted on unwilling patients.[10] In the postwar years, a large number of state prison systems and institutions within the federal system housed ongoing therapeutic and experimental research programs. These programs were "considered acceptable and even praiseworthy, since malaria was a serious threat to our military men during the war, and the research project afforded the prisoners an opportunity to contribute to the war effort."[11] Through their participation, white prisoners were able to enact their citizenship in ways that were denied to black prisoners. Black prisoners' lesser participation was linked to their lesser status as citizens; they could not be real patriots, sacrificing their bodies for the sake of the nation. Perhaps the whiteness of prisoner subjects enabled the effort to construct the testing program as patriotic, as one that, if allowed to be carried out without further government regulation, would strengthen the nation by speeding up technoscientific process and shoring up U.S. hegemony.

A CIVIC DUTY TO CONTRIBUTE

During and after World War II, a discourse of ethics, justice, and citizenship framed the pervasive yet contentious practice of drug testing in U.S. prisons. This research enterprise became a patriotic one, in which prisoners could understand their participation in drug experiments as contributing to the nation's war effort. Drug companies touted participation in drug testing as a way for prisoners to realize and expand their rights and responsibilities as citizens. This scientific program also became interpreted through new ethical frameworks that sidestepped international ethics norms to justify the use of prisoners as subjects in experimental biomedical research.

In the years following the Nuremberg doctors' trial and the articulation of the set of research ethics principles known as the Nuremberg Code, the world's leading medical professional groups, including the American Medical Association and the World Medical Association, revised their codes of conduct to state explicitly that it is unethical for prisoners to participate in medical experiments.[12] Paradoxically, these pronouncements preceded the most expansive growth of prison drug testing programs in U.S. carceral history. One of the key features of the Nazi experiments that qualified them as war crimes was that the human subjects involved could not freely choose to participate (or not) in the experiments. The indictment in the Nuremberg doctors' trial reads: "It was a part of the said common design, conspiracy, plans, and enterprises to perform medical experiments upon concentration camp inmates and other living human subjects, without their consent, in the course of which experiments the defendants committed the murders, brutalities, cruelties, tortures, atrocities, and other inhuman acts."[13] Forced internment creates a moral context in which people cannot exercise freedom of choice, and the absence of conditions that facilitate free choice makes for an unethical scientific practice. Voluntary consent is the first ethical principle that emerged out of the Nuremberg trials, one that continues to shape international norms for the conduct of ethical research involving human subjects. The Nuremberg Code cautions that "the voluntary consent of the human subject is absolutely essential."[14]

When questions about the ethics of medical experimentation on prisoners are applied to the Nazis, the answers are always consistent with Nazi Germany's position as modernity's ultimate moral failure: the Nazis were monsters who conducted the worst forms of scientific experimentation on humans. When questions about the ethics of medical experimentation on prisoners were applied to the treatment of prisoners in the United States in the postwar years, American exceptionalism tended to shape the responses.[15] The assumption of moral superiority attached to the United States defined the medical ethical frameworks applied to prisoners. Rebecca Lowen, who served as a consultant to the Advisory Committee on Human Radiation Experiments, established by President Bill Clinton in 1994, has observed that the moral debate within major medical journals between 1946 and 1963 was "largely defensive, stating the importance of human experimentation to the advancement of medical science, arguing that the behavior of Nazi doctors was a manifestation of the evil of totalitarianism rather than of human experimentation, and claiming that the United States' purported democratic culture ensured that human experimentation in the U.S. would be unlikely to pose ethical or moral problems."[16]

The moral contradictions that shaped the different frameworks applied to each nation-state were made apparent when one of the Nazi physicians on trial for exposing concentration camp detainees to malaria gave a nod to the U.S. doctors doing the same work in Statesville Penitentiary (Illinois), who gave the Nazis the idea for their research.[17] Both prior to and after the Nuremberg trials, it was standard practice, and considered ethical, to subject U.S. prisoners to medical experiments. In fact, the United States demanded the removal of a provision in a 1961 draft of a new international code of ethics on human experimentation that stated that "persons retained in prisons, penitentiaries, or reformatories—being 'captive groups'—should not be used as subjects of experiment."[18] This code of ethics would later be affirmed as the Helsinki Declaration of 1966, a second major articulation of ethical research norms.

The immoral and inhumane practices of closed institutions like prisons are understood to be immoral and inhumane only when they become publicly visible; prior to their exposure to light, they are accepted as perfectly rational, normalized, and humane. Eventually, concerned politicians, doctors, and journalists began to raise serious questions about the ethics and morality of drug testing in American prisons.[19] Doctors like Irving Ladimer, Henry Beecher, and Maurice Pappworth wrote essays critical of the practice in prominent medical journals.[20] Jessica Mitford, an investigative journalist in the muckraking tradition, authored the landmark 1973 text *Kind and Usual Punishment: The Prison Business*. Her indictment of "the prison business" and its deep connections to corporate and academic interests was published during a pivotal moment, when efforts were being made to examine and, at least potentially, reform American imprisonment. Because her research was conducted during a period when scholars, journalists, and citizens in general had comparatively greater access to prisons than they do now, and because the publication of her book itself led prisons to close themselves off more completely from outsiders (for fear that their unjust and unethical practices would be exposed), Mitford's work stands alone in the body of prison muckraking journalism for its proximity to the social practices that take place behind prison walls. Mitford's view was that prisons used a cloak of secrecy to control the flow of information about their relationships to drug companies, government agencies, and academic researchers.

Exposés like Mitford's led to the passage of the National Research Act of 1974, which created the National Commission for the Protection of Human Subjects of Biomedical and Behavioral Research.[21] The commission held congressional hearings, conducted site visits of institutions where research on prisoners was ongoing, and conducted extensive original research on biomedical research programs in the United States. The commission is best known for authoring *The Belmont Report,* published in 1979, which spurred the implementation of institutional review boards and new modes of conducting ethical reviews of biomedical and behavioral research in the United States.[22] Based on the commission's findings, the federal government moved to establish new legal protections for all people, but especially prisoners, participating in any research on human subjects. New federal regulations adopted in 1980 restricted the types of research for which prisoners could serve as subjects to four categories: (1) research on the possible effects, causes, and processes of incarceration and/or criminal behavior; (2) research on prisons as institutional structures or prisoners as incarcerated persons; (3) research on conditions that particularly affect prisoners as a class; and (4) research developed to improve prisoners' health and well-being.

In anticipation of and opposition to the recommendations of the National Commission for the Protection of Human Subjects, the pharmaceutical industry tried to preempt the eventual curtailment of drug testing in prisons. Drug companies argued that current regulatory frameworks were adequate to ensure that drug testing using prisoners was being conducted in an ethical manner and that further regulation of their activities would stall advances in drug research and development. Despite concerns among many ethicists about prisoners' capacity to exercise free and informed consent, drug corporations selfishly asserted that the exclusion of prisoners from pharmaceutical research was an abrogation of prisoners' "right" to make a contribution to American society and technoscientific progress. Late in the summer of 1973, the

Pharmaceutical Manufacturers Association and the National Council on Crime and Delinquency cosponsored a conference titled "Prisons, Inmates, and Drug Testing," at which participants interested in drug research in state and federal prisons would "review the important issues with responsible representatives from a cross-section of involved groups." Attended by drug researchers, corporate executives, ex-prisoners, correctional officials, government officials, and civil rights advocates, this "balanced and reasoned" conference was represented as a response to the "relatively sensational" media reports about drug testing and other biomedical exploitations in American society in the early 1970s. The hope of the conveners was that the conference attendees would develop a set of guidelines that would "ensure a higher ethical standard in the conduct of drug studies in prisons."[23] The "key issues" addressed at the conference were framed as a set of questions that seemed to presuppose their own answers:

1. Do we want a continuation of the high rate of therapeutic progress which has characterized the past quarter century?
2. Are we in danger, through an excess of regulation, of bringing an end to significant drug research in the United States?
3. Is continued drug research a contribution or an obstruction to prison reform?
4. Can drug research contribute to an expansion of the rights of prisoners?
5. Under what circumstances can an inmate volunteer, with a minimum of coercion, as a subject in a drug study?
6. Can we regulate researchers to ensure adherence to a high standard of ethics?[24]

Of course, it is not surprising that the drug companies pushed back against increased regulation and lobbied for conditions that would make it easier for them to conduct experiments on prisoners. We would expect that drug companies would advocate for continuing the practices that benefited them directly, and that they would frame those benefits as ones in which the citizenry might share equally.

The drug companies sought to distinguish drug testing programs in prisons from the "horror stories" that had circulated about biomedical experimentation in prisons involving such methods as psychosurgery and behavior modification. Framing drug testing as "relatively low-risk and well-regulated," the authors of the summary report of the conference challenged further regulation of drug research: "Another serious problem is that drug research is already controlled in the United States by detailed regulations, and unfortunately, further *improvement* in the protection and controls surrounding drug studies would tend to increase this burden."[25] In a brief section titled "The Need for Therapeutic Progress," they pressed for the continuation of "the extraordinary record of the past three decades" in drug research and development and lamented the scrutiny applied to their work. They made a utilitarian moral argument, suggesting that if we all want to experience the benefits that biomedical progress manifests (like drugs for cancer and heart disease), we must not question the "relatively low risk" of suffering by the few prisoners used as subjects for experimentation. They wrote:

> Some seriously question whether further therapeutic progress is necessary in view of the attendant risks. The findings of this inquiry are based on the convictions that the continued good health of our nation and the continued high standards of excellence of medicine in the U.S. today depend upon maintaining *creative* drug research in the U.S. However, it is a characteristic of our times that everything is scrutinized and questioned. We are not automatically assured of a continuation of our past rate of achievement in therapeutic progress. Excessive government scrutiny, regulation, and review can destroy the opportunities and incentives upon which significant drug research is based. If the public ceases to value therapeutic progress, if in the pursuit of other values, we destroy the climate within which research flourishes, significant drug research will cease in the U.S.[26]

Excluding prisoners as subjects in drug studies would require, in their words, "major changes in the procedures for satisfying Phase One regulatory requirements."[27]

What is surprising are the moral and civic arguments the authors advanced regarding the benefits to prisoners of participating in drug research. The overarching argument that drug companies made sought to tie prisoners' participation in drug trials to civic/patriotic duty and rights. The authors asserted that "the benefits for participants in research include: better health care, wages, and the opportunity to make decisions and participate in something of benefit to mankind."[28] Further, they claimed, "Inmates benefit from better medical care, contact with people outside the correctional system, an opportunity to learn about research, feelings of self-worth resulting from participation in research, and contributions to the inmates' welfare fund, as well as improvements to facilities."[29]

The authors argued that prisoners should be able to continue to volunteer to be research subjects in drug studies because this would give them increased access to medical care (a morally good thing), higher wages (an economically good thing), and the ability to exercise free choice to help others (a rational civic duty). This last argument seemed especially important for the conference attendees in the work group on ethics, rights, and laws. They postulated that the "inmate is given an important opportunity to exercise responsibility for his actions when he is allowed to make a personal decision about participation in research—an opportunity otherwise lacking in the prison environment."[30]

These arguments about the theoretical benefits to inmates who participate in drug research sidestepped the more fundamental moral question about the use of prisoners in any kind of research outlined by the Nuremberg Code. The conference attendees recognized that prisoners are "in a particularly powerless position to protect their own rights," and yet "Phase One studies can offer important opportunities for inmates to exercise their rights and to assume some control over their lives."[31] Amazingly, they framed participation in drug studies as a right to which prisoners are entitled, with the denial of that opportunity therefore representing an abrogation of their rights. The critical "rights" question—that is, whether or not prisoners are able to exercise free choice to volunteer in drug research—remained unresolved at the conference, as stated repeatedly in the summary report:

> It could not be resolved whether it is possible for an inmate to make a truly free choice in prison.

> Though the degree to which an inmate can freely volunteer under the conditions of prison life is debated, that concern was not felt to be sufficient justification to discontinue drug research in prisons.

> The question whether an inmate can truly volunteer was not answered; the group took a more practical approach by defining a volunteer as one who consents by signing the consent form.[32]

Parke, Davis and Company (also known as Parke-Davis), one of the major drug corporations involved in extensive prison research, developed a new human subjects policy in 1975. What is most relevant about this policy for this discussion is the doublespeak embedded in the policy text: the company will respect and safeguard the health and rights of research subjects by not respecting or safeguarding the health and rights of research subjects as outlined in the Nuremburg Code. The "Policy on the Use of Humans as Subjects in Clinical Investigation in an Institutional Setting" reads:

> It is the policy of Parke, Davis & Company (Parke-Davis) to respect and safeguard the health and rights of all individuals who may be used as subjects in clinical investigation in institutional settings. In the conduct of its clinical investigation, this company's action will conform with the ten principles known as the Nuremberg Code . . . to the extent that they or their basic objectivities are applicable literally or in principle, and other applicable codes to the extent that they are not in conflict with the Nuremberg Code.[33]

In a policy statement provided to the National Commission for the Protection of Human Subjects, the PMA outlined a nearly identical set of guiding principles for drug companies that sponsor or conduct drug research in prisons. This statement begins with the dual recognition of "the need to preserve the ethical and legal rights of prisoners" and "the contribution that prison testing has made to medical progress."[34] The PMA argued that prisoners were desirable research subjects for phase 1 and bioavailability studies because of the need for close supervision and monitoring of these subjects and their responses to drug compounds under similar environmental conditions, such as diet and work habits. According to the PMA, not only are prisoners ideal subjects in a scientific sense, but also participation in drug research translates into social and civic benefits for both the prisoners and society:

> It is abundantly clear that well-controlled studies can be and are conducted in such institutions which contribute to the social rehabilitation of the prisoner, with maximum safety, and with apparent benefits to both inmates and society at large. Indeed, a cogent argument can be made for preserving the prisoner's right to participate in research programs, under appropriate safeguards, as one of the few rights left to the incarcerated individual.[35]

Strangely, no U.S. court has ever affirmed a "right" of citizens to participate as subjects in research, a legal question that remains unresolved in U.S. law. Citing a 1944 U.S. circuit court ruling that found that a prisoner "retains all the rights of an ordinary citizen except those expressly, or by necessary implication, taken away from him by law," the staff of the National Commission for the Protection of Human Subjects also had difficulty answering this legal question.[36]

In the mid-1970s, the PMA and its member companies lost the policy argument about using prisoners as subjects in drug testing programs. One year after *The Belmont Report* was published, the recommendations of the National Commission for the Protection of Human Subjects were translated into federal regulations (as mentioned earlier), and prison drug testing programs were shut down entirely by 1980. However, the moral arguments made in support of using prisoners as test subjects, which were grounded in a discourse of ethics, justice, and citizenship, lay dormant, waiting for the right opportunity to resurface.

THE RACIAL BIOPOLITICS OF PARTICIPATION

In the mid- to late 1970s, a one-way interpretation of racism dominated prisoner advocates' readings of the relationship between race and drug testing programs. This interpretation held that the only way in which drug testing programs could be racist was if black prisoners were enrolled in drug studies in higher numbers than white prisoners, or if black prisoners were exposed to studies with higher risks than whites.[37] This interpretation was based on the fact that black prisoners outnumbered whites in many jurisdictions—it was simply the next logical step to assume that they would be recruited into drug studies in greater numbers. The members of the National Minority Conference on Human Experimentation, a subset of the National Commission for the Protection of Human Subjects, made this logical step in their summary as part of the work of the larger commission:

> Since there is a disproportionate Third World representation in prisons today, it is agreed that the issue of prisoners and race are merged. It is unethical to ask minority prisoners to bear the greater portion of risk when benefitting society at large. Any required risks should be evenly distributed in the prison society itself as well as among all ethnic groups in society.[38]

Somewhat paradoxically, the available evidence suggests that the assumption of black overrepresentation in prison drug studies is contestable. On one side of this equation, you have Harriet Washington and Allen Hornblum, who argue that black prisoners were subjects in greater proportion to their numbers in the noninstitutionalized population. On the other side, you have Jon Harkness and the National Commission for the Protection of Human Subjects, who argue that *among prison populations,* white prisoners outnumbered prisoners of color in drug studies. The evidence suggests that white prisoners were enrolled in prison drug studies in higher numbers than were black prisoners, although there is no publicly available information as to whether or not black prisoners were disproportionately enrolled in studies that were riskier.

In the only empirical analysis conducted of the racial representativeness of drug study populations, carried out during a site visit to the State Prison at Southern Michigan at Jackson in November 1975 (which I will discuss again in a moment), the National Commission for the Protection of Human Subjects found that

> although blacks comprise almost 68% of the nonsubject prison population, they are only about 31% of the subject pool. (Data furnished to the Commission by Dr. William Woodward of the University of Maryland showed a similar inverted racial pattern in the biomedical research program at the Maryland House of Corrections at Jessup.)[39]

Furthermore, the interpretation that racism required black overrepresentation in drug trials was also misleading. As Jon Harkness, the lone historian of prison drug studies, states:

> In racial terms, discrimination against African-American prisoners led to an underrepresentation of black prisoners in prison-based experiments. In the 1970s, some activists—failing to recognize this inversion—managed to combine the disproportionately high number of African Americans in prison with the stark racial exploitation of the well-known Syphilis Study to construe experimentation on prisoners as a racial issue in a politically potent—but erroneous fashion.[40]

Unfortunately, Harkness's analysis of racism more or less begins and ends with this claim in the first few pages of his unpublished, yet still highly respected, PhD dissertation.

Black underrepresentation in drug studies was structured by racism, given the concrete benefits attached to volunteering for studies, but not in the pattern that was evidenced in other forms of biomedical experimentation. It is difficult (if not entirely impossible) to generalize about the research practices in the dozens of prisons around the country where drug studies were carried out, but inmates who participated were usually given access to extensive health screenings and medical treatment.[41] Prior to the 1976 U.S. Supreme Court decision in *Estelle v. Gamble*, prisons were not required to provide basic medical care to prisoners during their incarceration. Prisoner test subjects also were given a break from the monotony and dangers of routinized prison life.[42] It was a privilege, in a specific sense, to participate, to be included, as a subject in a drug study. There was also the not small issue of monetary compensation, the reason most prisoner subjects participated in drug studies.[43] Prisoners earned cash per procedure, per study, often linked to the duration of their participation. This money conferred a sense of security and protection, and so perhaps improved their mental health. Based on this interpretation, biopower affected the distribution of valued resources by granting white prisoners greater access to material goods that directly or indirectly improved health, not necessarily by exposing black prisoners to the dangers of the drug testing programs.

In the early 1970s, Mary Lee Bundy, a fierce advocate for the active generation of information that can lead to human liberation and professor in the College of Library and Information Sciences at the University of Maryland in College Park, started an organization called Urban Information Interpreters with some of her colleagues. Bundy instructed the group to study the racial dynamics within a drug testing program at the Maryland House of Correction at Jessup. Urban Information Interpreters joined with several other organizations in this effort, including the Black Student Union of the University of Maryland, the American Civil Liberties Union's National Prison Project, and the National Conference of Black Lawyers. Established in 1959 under the aegis of the University of Maryland School of Medicine, and with funding from the U.S. Department of Defense, the National Institutes of Health, the FDA, and pharmaceutical firms, the Infectious Disease Area (IDA) at the Jessup facility served as an experimental unit within the prison for the evaluation of the effectiveness of vaccines "against certain infections such as typhoid fever, bacillary dysentery, cholera and other diarrheal diseases as well as influenza and the common cold."[44]

The collaborating organizations worked tirelessly to obtain information about this unit from state officials. The investigators wrote letters, made phone calls, and attempted to interview government officials who should have had direct or indirect knowledge of the research program at Jessup. All of the researchers' attempts to gain access to detailed information about the program and its central research findings were rebuffed. Ralph Williams, the warden of the House of Correction, replied in writing, "Thank you for your concern regarding activities of the Division of Correction and specifically, the Maryland House of Correction. However, much of the information you request is not subject to public disclosure, and, as such, I must unfortunately, deny same."

The secretive nature of prison drug testing programs makes it impossible to discern the national racial distribution of experimental patriots. Poor prison record keeping and the desire not to appear overtly racist undoubtedly account at least in part for the absence of racial knowledge about prison drug studies. The members of Urban Information Interpreters believed that knowledge of prison practices in general, as well as specific information regarding medical experimentation in prisons, exists in a closed system. Doctors and administrators retain control over the flow of information out of prisons so as to minimize or prevent public scrutiny. In 1974, Leslie Berger, a congressional staffer with Maryland representative Parren Mitchell, and Bundy wrote:

> Any program operating within a prison is automatically kept from public screening, for a prison is a system run by coercion and punitive control means, where as a matter of practice the public is not made privy to what goes on, and where inmate expression is habitually suppressed. Prison administrators characteristically seek to be the sole source of what the public is allowed to know about conditions inside. The failure on the part of the warden at Jessup to supply any information at all is a naked expression of this practice of withholding information from the public so as to protect the prison system from review and censure.[45]

Bundy and others connected to the prisoners' rights movement sought to illuminate racial injustices in the Maryland prison at Jessup, but they made a serious miscalculation when they made unsupported claims that black prisoners were being disproportionately exploited in the prison's drug testing program. With respect to the role of race in the program at Jessup the authors reasoned:

> It is difficult to say that IDA experiments are per se racist in nature; because both Black and White prisoners partake in them. However, it should be noted that the prison population ratio is eighty-to-ninety percent Black, in spite of quarterly fluctuations. But, for objectivity reasons, it is best that the reader makes his own inference.[46]

Without clear empirical evidence of racial disparities in rates of inclusion in the experiments, the authors were reluctant to claim that the program was in fact racist. Instead, they inferred from the fact that the prison population itself was predominantly black that the experimental subjects must be disproportionately black. I am not sure if they learned about the majority-white subjects in the Jessup experiments from the same physician who informed the National Commission for the Protection of Human Subjects of the pattern of "racial inversion" mentioned earlier. Nonetheless, once they determined that the experimental programs at Jessup were not racist in the way they had assumed, they continued to contest the broader program of experimentation at the prison, although now with more of a focus on the ethical complications of informed consent in prisons than on racial disproportionality.

For the National Commission for the Protection of Human Subjects, direct evidence of racial representation in prison drug trials was difficult, but not impossible, to unearth. Years earlier, in 1963, Parke-Davis and Upjohn Corporation joined together to conduct drug testing at the State Prison of Southern Michigan at Jackson. The state of Michigan permitted Parke-Davis and Upjohn to build a new 11,000-square-foot research facility on the grounds of the prison, which was, at that time, the largest prison in the United States, in both physical size and population. As part of its inquiry, the National Commission received extensive documentation from Parke-Davis that chronicled the drug protocols the company carried out in this facility from 1969 through 1974, including a number of studies of unnamed psychotropic drugs. Unfortunately, the documentation did not discuss these studies in any detail. However, in one interoffice memo dated January 1975, Parke-Davis's director of clinical pharmacology, T. C. Smith, reported to another administrator, G. D. Wood, the number and racial makeup of volunteers and active male participants in the studies for 1974. To my knowledge, this is the only publicly available corporate document that identifies the racial distribution of subjects in any prison drug testing program. The memo shows that "Negroid" prisoners who wished to gain acceptance into the drug testing protocol in 1974 had the lowest rate of acceptance for any measured racial group (36.4 percent, 82 prisoners), followed by "American Indian" (44.4 percent, 4 prisoners), "Caucasian" (45.2 percent, 187 prisoners), and "Mexican-American" prisoners (53.9 percent, 7 prisoners). In terms of the overall testing program that year, there were 394 "Caucasian" male prisoners (59.5 percent of the total), followed by 242 "Negroid" prisoners (36.5 percent of the total), 19 "Mexican-American" prisoners (2.9 percent of the total), and 7 "American Indian" prisoners (1.1 percent of the total). These numbers did not include the prisoners in the Upjohn studies that year, nor were the prisoner totals for any other year noted. But the memo notes that as of November 1975, there were five active research protocols at the State Prison of Southern Michigan, including two tolerance studies, one for an unknown tranquilizer (Protocol 683-41) and the other for an antidepressant (Protocol 781-2 and 781-3), with twelve subjects each.[47]

As a biopolitical program, prison drug testing constituted a racist structure by unfairly targeting and benefiting white prisoners and by targeting and exploiting black prisoners. Biopower confers upon favored groups an investment in life, an increase in exposure to the social conditions that improve health and foster vitality. Because race identifies populations who have access to the investments in health that flow from what institutions do, we have to consider how race functions not only to justify the deaths of internal enemies but also to improve the lives of favored populations. Even in these prison drug studies, biopower and race function to privilege white men, in this case increasing health investments reserved for the prisoners who participated in drug experiments while at the same time excluding "Negroid" male prisoners. In truth, all of these prisoners, regardless of their racial group membership, were subjected to clinical research that in my view was unethical and inhumane on its face. Thankfully, to some degree, that was then. What about now?

In 2006, the Institute of Medicine released a controversial report titled *Ethical Considerations for Research Involving Prisoners,* which revisited and proposed changes to the ethical and regulatory frameworks that have outlawed prison drug testing programs since 1980. The IOM committee responsible for the report had four mandates: (1) to consider whether the ethical bases for research with prisoners differ from those for research with nonprisoners; (2) to develop an ethical framework for the conduct of research with prisoners; (3) to identify, based on the ethical framework developed, considerations or safeguards necessary to ensure that research with prisoners is conducted ethically; and (4) to identify issues and needs for future consideration and study.[48] Yes, the IOM considered whether to restart prison drug testing programs in our time.

In justifying the IOM's reconsideration of the recommendations of the National Commission for the Protection of Human Subjects,

Lawrence Gostin, the committee chair, argued that research involving prisoners can "afford great benefits" such as "help[ing] policy makers to make correctional settings more humane and effective in achieving legitimate social goals such as deterrence and rehabilitation" and "help[ing] policy makers better understand and respond to the myriad health problems faced by prisoners."[49] Of course, prisoners' wishes matter, too: "If a prisoner wants to participate in research, his or her views ought to be taken into account."[50] In what moral universe is the IOM functioning? How can it justify placing a new "research burden" on imprisoned citizens? Whose interests are advanced by permitting new access to prison populations?

Opponents of the IOM's recommendations have argued against the dismantling of the categorical system of review because they view it as reopening U.S. prisons to biomedical and pharmaceutical interests.[51] This shifting ethical framework affirms the notion of prisoners' presumed rights to participate in drug testing as long as they stand to benefit from such research without being exposed to undue harms—a foundational principle of the Nuremburg Code and contemporary human subjects research. Yet these arguments position medical advances and the overarching social good as highly valued outcomes of prison drug testing, in direct contradiction to the eighth principle of the Helsinki Declaration.[52]

Even now, drug companies' interests continue to define the moral and ethical terms under which prisoners are used as experimental patriots. Yet, according to the IOM, "today, it is impossible to know how many prisoners are involved in [any biomedical or behavioral] studies because no central database exists of such information."[53] And, as the Urban Information Interpreters argued forty years ago, government secrecy complicates efforts to document unfair practices linked to capitalist exploitation in prison contexts:

> Secrecy, if not in this situation, then in others, permits doctors, drug companies and others in their hire to make enormous profit from the exploitation of incarcerated people. . . . The real significance of government secrecy is the very real role it plays in the systematic exploitation of people.[54]

Unknown and uncounted imprisoned men have paid with their brains and bodies to advance technoscientific progress and biomedical knowledge and to increase corporate profits. This perverse system of racial beneficence may have unfairly benefited white male prisoners for years while simultaneously targeting black bodies with dangerous science, as was done in so-called free society.

Decades of unfettered access to prisons as testing sites for drug studies helped to position the pharmaceutical industry as among the most profitable industries in contemporary global capitalism. While prisons served as the repositories for a wide range of social and biomedical experimentation, prison bodies became one of the central sources of biomedical knowledge and profit generation for pharmaceutical companies. As far as I know, there is no way to determine conclusively whether or not psychotropics approved before 1980 were tested on U.S. prisoners before they were unleashed on the general population. In all likelihood, prisoners constituted an important clinical population for the study of psychotropics in this period. Drug companies were not required to disclose whether their test subjects were prisoners during the FDA drug approval process. Moreover, the researchers who published the clinical trial data from those studies were not required to disclose that information in medical journals. Perhaps that was just how things were done back then. And, as we have learned, powerful interests would like us to go back to the way things were. We know that the U.S. pharmaceutical industry got a big head start by relying on prison bodies as research subjects, and because of that great, cheap start, they were well positioned to push pharmaceuticals out into the world. In the next chapter, I turn to discussion of the broader U.S. carceral state, where psychotropics intersect with the hard realities and heavy burdens of psychic trauma, unequal protection under the law, and the ethics of care.

FOUR

PSYCHIC STATES OF EMERGENCY

The Pacification of Institutional Crises

On September 12, 2014, Kamilah Brock, a black woman who worked as a banker in New York City, was stopped in her car, a 2003 BMW, by New York police officers, purportedly because she did not have her hands on the steering wheel while she was listening and dancing to music when stopped at a red light.[1] The officers detained her for several hours, without filing any charges, and impounded her car. The next night, Brock returned to the local police precinct station to retrieve her car. According to the complaint she subsequently filed in the U.S. District Court for the Southern District of New York, officers at the station "did not provide [Brock] with any guidance [about her car], but rather with insults, condescension, and disbelief that she owned a BMW."[2] Shockingly, instead of helping Brock get her car back, the police handcuffed her, called an ambulance, and had her transported to the local public hospital, Harlem Hospital, labeling her "an emotionally disturbed person." Then, as if the situation were not bad enough, upon her arrival at the hospital, Brock was handcuffed to a gurney and forcibly injected with lorazepam and lithium, two psychotropic drugs, without her consent. Despite her pleas that she did not need any mental health treatment, hospital psychiatrists issued evaluations that "were the direct cause of her confinement" at Harlem Hospital, where she would remain, against her will, for eight days. Adding insult to injury, after she was released on September 22, she was sent a bill for her hospital stay: $13,637.

Rolling in her BMW, Kamilah Brock challenged the bedrock assumptions that uphold white supremacist capitalist patriarchy, which demand that black people, especially black women, be subservient, poor, and submissive. Yet there she was—an economically successful and free black woman with a lively spirit. For challenging those assumptions, Brock was subjected to two of the government's most potent weapons for putting people like her back in their place: involuntary civil commitment and forced psychotropic drugging. Ostensibly free U.S. citizens, like Brock, have the right to protest in court if they are subjected to forced commitment and forced psychotropic drugging. And they have the right to sue for damages stemming from such treatment, should they have the good fortune of being released, a right that Brock exercised in this case. However, the ability to exercise these rights is unequally distributed across people who experience the misfortune of being held in custody by the state. Brock's jailers overdosed on the power the state had given them to take people into custody and drug them without their consent, a power that is disproportionately used to commit black people like Brock to mental health facilities in the United States.

As this story suggests, the government wields the authority to hold people in custody and administer psychotropic drugs at will. The government can use its power of *parens patriae* to place people in custody under the rhetoric of "care," or it can use its police power to hold people it deems to be dangerous to others.[3] Holding people in custody is legally justified within a *state of emergency,* a supposedly temporary crisis state in which the laws that govern a society are suspended so that the government can defend itself against existential threats; examples of such threats are epidemics, civil war, and invasion. Political theorist Giorgio Agamben uses the term "states of exception" for those situations in which the suspension of the rule of law, rather than being temporary, becomes a permanent form of government.[4]

Drawing on this idea, the stories I relate in this chapter unfold in *psychic states of emergency*—institutional crises that are used to justify custodial power, the power to hold bodies and, within them, use psychotropics to transform brains for the purpose of managing vulnerable populations. Psychic states of emergency work by effectively dissolving the thin boundary between therapeutic medical practice, in which people can freely choose to participate, and coercive state violence, which people cannot legally refuse. Thus far in this book I have focused on prisoners, who certainly exist within this space. Their transgression of the law opens them to treatment *as* punishment, a distinction without a difference when it comes to the administration of psychotropic drugs.

I have examined how psychotropics serve to prop up unjust laws and policies that produce mass confinement, and I have been trying to figure out if the United States could dump 2.2 million people into the prison–industrial complex without the use of psychotropics as chemical restraints. In the process, I have learned about troubling patterns of psychotropic use in other prison-like carceral institutions. As I explained in my Introduction, I use the term *captive America* to refer to the U.S. carceral state, the web of government-run institutions that hold people in various forms of custody. Think beyond prisons to nursing homes, the military, and the foster care system. As a society, we have given these custodial institutions special legal powers to hold and mold large groups of people by nearly any means necessary. These are all social institutions in which people live and work for long periods of time. If it is impossible to know exactly how psychotropic drugs are used within prisons, perhaps by tracing their use elsewhere in U.S. society we can begin to understand how these drugs are used to put people in their place (and keep them there). How do psychotropics uphold mass confinement in a pervasive and dangerous way that is really about keeping a lid on institutions, and a society, in crisis?

PSYCHOTROPICS AND THE PROCESS OF DEINSTITUTIONALIZATION

In the context of mental health, the creation of the current U.S. carceral state and the institutional crises that flow from it began with the closure of state psychiatric hospitals, a process that saw more than 400,000 people released back into U.S. society beginning in the 1940s. When the first prescription psychotropic drug, Thorazine, was approved by the U.S. Food and Drug Administration in 1954, the mass migration of hundreds of thousands of mentally ill people out of state psychiatric hospitals and into other total institutions, like prisons, was well under way.[5] While drug companies, hospital staff, and mental health policy makers heralded the great therapeutic transformation that antipsychotic drugs represented at the policy level, the introduction and rapid diffusion of these drugs into state psychiatric hospitals in the mid-1950s did not actually lead to significant increases in hospital discharges.[6] Rather, psychotropic drugs such as antipsychotics entered the context of mental health system reform in the United States right at the moment when the state psychiatric hospital system was about to collapse. According to E. Fuller Torrey, a prominent mental health expert, antipsychotics may not have "started the engine" of deinstitutionalization, but they "provided the fuel that initially made it run."[7] Psychotropic drugs may not have "opened the back door" of the state psychiatric hospitals, but they kept that door open by providing a means through which mental illness could be humanely treated in community settings. More important, psychotropics followed mental illness out the back door of the asylum and in through the front doors of other total institutional settings, where they currently constitute the principal treatment modality for people living with psychic distress.[8]

The failure to establish community mental health centers across the country, coupled with the nation's decision to close the great majority of state mental hospitals, created a permanent institutional crisis for hundreds of thousands of people.[9] The closure of state psychiatric hospitals generated a number of unintended consequences for other social institutions that already served populations experiencing distress. While outpatient mental health care provided some relief for milder cases of disorder in community settings, facilities that still provided custodial care constituted a patchwork network of total institutions that could receive more severely impaired populations.[10] The movement of mentally ill people from state hospitals to other social institutions has been termed *transinstitutionalization,* which Carol Warren defines as "the transfer of mental patients, juveniles, and the elderly from facilities funded by state and county to facilities organized by entrepreneurs who provide beds, food, and clothing from the various types of welfare payment received by clientele and/or from insurance plans."[11] Transinstitutionalization represents a cyclical effort to shift the financial and political responsibility for mentally ill people from state-level institutions to federal and private institutions and back again.[12]

The process of deinstitutionalization not only had the effect of growing the populations of the mentally ill in nursing homes, jails, and prisons directly, but it also created a context in which these total institutions would later become linked, this time indirectly, to one another in new ways that would converge around the widespread use of psychotropics. As people have flowed from one institutional context to another, with few viable alternative therapies in place, psychotropics have followed them—into the prison, as I have described, but also into the military, the nursing home, and the youth foster system. While the availability of new psychotropics in the 1950s did not initiate the process of deinstitutionalization, psychotropics certainly made it possible for mental health care providers to treat a range of psychic traumas in settings outside psychiatric hospitals.

In addition to these challenges, politicians and community groups have pressed for regulatory reforms and oversight mechanisms for social groups that are particularly vulnerable to psychic trauma and live within this network of custody. Consider the string of congressional hearings that have focused on the linkages between psychotropics and vulnerable groups. Congress first held hearings on the role played by psychotropics in the process of the deinstitutionalization of state psychiatric hospitals in 1994.[13] The Omnibus Budget Reconciliation Act of 1987 included regulations concerning the distribution of antipsychotic drugs to elders living in nursing homes; this had the intended effect of lowering antipsychotic use among seniors, but it also had the unintended effect of increasing antidepressant use in this population.[14] In 2008, a congressional hearing was held to examine the excessive use of psychotropics among children in foster care. At that hearing, Misty Stenslie, a professional social worker and foster mother who had spent her own childhood in the foster care system, was asked why she thought so many youth in foster care are prescribed psychotropic drugs. She replied:

> So we do a lot of things in child welfare to try to make things easier for the adults [who run and work in the system]; and, so, I think a lot of times managing a young person's behavior through the use of medication is a way to try to make it possible for foster parents to stick with this kid just a little longer, or for the group home not to send them to a higher level of care, that we do it so the adults in their lives can figure out how to cope with them.
>
> I think that a lot of times medication is used as a chemical restraint for children whose behavior gets out of control.[15]

Finally, consider the more recent congressional attention focused on the high rates of suicide among active-duty military members and veterans, and the potential connection of psychotropics to these suicides.[16] The institutional crises chronicled in this chapter are linked together by the reliance on psychotropics to manage the flow of people in and out of state custody.

MAKING MINDLESS WAR ENDLESS
The practice of soldiers taking a little something to help them manage the psychic trauma of war is not new, but the use of psychotropics in the activity-duty military is a relatively recent development.[17] In the

long aftermath of 9/11, U.S. troops have been deployed to conduct war operations in Afghanistan, Iraq, and elsewhere around the world. In the so-called War on Terror, soldiers are exposed to endless traumas and high levels of stress in combat zones. Unlike in any prior conflict, psychotropics are used to alleviate or control insomnia, anxiety, nerves, and symptoms of posttraumatic stress disorder (PTSD). Although estimates of the numbers of active-duty soldiers taking psychotropics vary, a June 2010 report from the Defense Department's Pharmacoeconomic Center noted that 213,972 (or around 20 percent) of the 1.1 million active-duty troops surveyed were taking some type of psychotropic drug in the form of antidepressants, antipsychotics, sedative hypnotics, or other controlled substances.[18] In the words of military officials, psychotropics are openly deployed in combat zones to "conserve fighting strength" and to "enhance performance."[19]

Here's what happened. In 2001, the Department of Defense changed its long-standing Central Command policy forbidding the use of psychotropics by active-duty military, and military psychiatrists began distributing these drugs to soldiers to help them manage the traumatic stress of war, with the goal of keeping them ready for future deployment.[20] The revised policy allows troops a 90- or 180-day supply of any psychotropic drugs included in the military's pharmacy formulary before they are deployed for combat. It has been reported that "drugs like Valium and Xanax, used to treat depression, [and] the antipsychotic Seroquel, originally developed to treat schizophrenia, bipolar disorders, mania and depression" all appear in the military's formulary.[21] One of the reasons for this policy shift was that criticism had arisen because military doctors were found to be prescribing medications, especially for pain management, at rates much lower than those of civilian doctors.[22]

According to reporting by the *Austin American-Statesman* newspaper, the Defense Logistics Agency, which is tasked with logistics support for the military, spent $2.7 billion on antidepressants between 2002 and 2012.[23] From 2005 to 2011 there was a 76 percent increase in all psychotropics prescribed to active-duty troops: orders for antipsychotics increased by 200 percent, antianxiety drugs by 170 percent, antiepileptics by 70 percent, and antidepressants by 40 percent.[24] Michael Knowlan and his colleagues surveyed 732 naval physicians regarding their current use of and attitudes toward prescribing psychotropics for deployable personnel. They found that some of the physicians supported the continued use of SSRIs by active-duty troops because, compared with older types of drugs, SSRIs are seen as relatively harmless and highly effective in managing combat stress.[25]

The military defends this practice by asserting that while prescribing these drugs involves calculated risks, it is necessary because many service members face multiple deployments. As the inability to continue in military service has become an increasingly significant issue over the past two decades because of the psychic trauma that soldiers experience, military officials have sought to reserve the right to administer psychotropics involuntarily. William Grant and Phillip Resnick examined the development of federal laws and constitutional principles that inform court decisions regarding soldiers' right to refuse treatment of psychotropic medication. These practices, which may include involuntary hospitalization, could be linked to military officials' desire to expedite the return of troops to active duty. At the time of their study, Grant and Resnick found there were no protocols for the treatment of soldiers through involuntary administration of psychotropics and hospitalization.[26]

High rates of psychotropic use and their effects on soldiers' bodies have been linked to increases in suicide and violent behavior, including sexual assault and violence.[27] According to the FDA, all antidepressants must carry warnings on their labels stating that young adults (up to the age of twenty-four) have shown an increased risk of suicide when taking these drugs in short-term, controlled clinical trials. In 2012, the Associated Press reported that there had been 349 suicides among active-duty military personnel that year, more than the 295 killed in action in Afghanistan during the same period.[28] By 2014, soldier suicides were averaging twenty per day and accounted for 18 percent of all suicides in the United States.[29]

Critics also point to issues such as soldiers being deployed with enough medication for 180 days, much longer than the common six-week clinical trial, and soldiers' ability to trade medications freely among themselves. The practice of deploying soldiers with large quantities of psychotropics at their disposal has allowed troops to stockpile medications, a common reason for overdoses and inappropriate drug switching or trading.[30] Further, because active-duty soldiers often spend extended periods on the battlefield, it is difficult for doctors to schedule follow-up appointments with them, or to monitor the effects of these drugs. Not only are overmedication and lack of follow-up serious problems,

but also many soldiers are prescribed several drugs at one time (a practice known as polypharmacy), which may be dangerous because little
is known about how some psychotropics interact with each other, especially over the long term. Recognizing the possibilities for harm associated with psychotropics, some military bases have instituted drug
"give back" days, when soldiers can return unused medications. Also,
doctors on some bases have extended their therapy programs to include
different kinds of treatments rather than relying on drugs alone; some
of these have proven effective in alleviating the symptoms of PTSD.
However, while strategies like "exposure therapy" may be effective, for
many soldiers, both access to psychiatric help and the desire to seek
such help may be limited.[31]

In addition to the fact that there is a shortage of trained psychiatrists available to active-duty troops, when soldiers are able to access
mental health treatment from military doctors, they face two issues:
the stigma associated with seeking treatment and the lack of any guarantee of patient privacy rights.[32] The Department of Defense reserves
the right to access the medical records of any member of the military
in a "need to know" situation, and exactly what constitutes need to
know is not defined.[33] This lack of ensured confidentiality inevitably
leads to some service members not seeking out military psychologists
or psychiatrists to address any mental health issues they may have, not
only because of the gendered expectations associated with masculine
behavior but also because being treated for psychological problems may
be detrimental to advancement within the military itself.[34] All of these
issues, taken together, may contribute to active-duty soldiers' relying
solely on psychotropics for their mental health needs.

It is unclear how the U.S. military is going to address its future
personnel needs against the backdrop of these issues related to mental health and psychotropic drug use. Perhaps a recent controversy can
shed some light on what the plan may be going forward. Historically,
the U.S. Army could seek a waiver and review for any recruit with a
history of serious mental health or drug use problems, so that the person could enlist. In 2009, a ban was placed on such waivers because of
the escalating crisis of suicides and other behavioral problems among
soldiers. Despite the ban, however, the army issued more than a thousand waivers between October 2016 and October 2017.[35] In November
2017, USA Today reported that the army was planning to end its ban on
waivers so that it could reach its target numbers for new recruits.[36] Days

later, the army clarified that it had no intention to end the waivers, but that it would be changing the process through which waivers are approved.[37] Clearly, the U.S. military understands that it has a population problem that is linked to mental health issues, violence, and suicide, some of which are endemic to conditions of perpetual war. It uses psychotropics as a major part of the solution to this crisis. The military is not the only custodial institution with a population problem, however.

ELDER ZOMBIE APOCALYPSE

In February 2018, Human Rights Watch published a landmark report titled *"They Want Docile": How Nursing Homes in the United States Overmedicate People with Dementia,* which describes what the organization learned from 109 visits and countless interviews in nursing homes around the country. Hundreds of people involved with nursing homes were interviewed, from staff to families to recognized medical experts. The report quotes the daughter of a seventy-five-year old Kansas woman who said that after the nursing home gave her mom an antipsychotic drug, she "would just sit there. . . . Just a zombie."[38] Currently, it is estimated that between 25 percent and 50 percent of nursing home residents are given psychotropic drugs.[39] It is becoming terrifyingly commonplace for elders to fear that they might end up as zombies in nursing homes. I have not studied such fears in my research for this book, but it seems that even cultural representations of nursing homes somehow always feature at least one elder, if not a roomful of elders, sitting or lying down, staring silently off into the distance, zombie-like.

This situation is not an accident but rather a consequence of the dislocations and economic deprivations that accompany late modern capitalism. Elders are admitted to nursing homes and assisted care facilities when their social needs and health problems have outpaced their families' ability to care for them. According to the 2012 *Nursing Home Data Compendium* (an annual publication of the U.S. government's Centers for Medicare and Medicaid Services), there were approximately 15,680 nursing home facilities in the United States in 2011, nearly three out of four of which were operated by for-profit companies. Nearly 1.5 million elders were living in U.S. nursing homes, and more than 750,000 were living in other types of residential institutions. Women made up nearly two-thirds of the 2012 nursing home population, and three out of four elders living in these institutions were white.[40]

By the late 1980s, the abuse of antipsychotic drugs in nursing homes in the United States had become so rampant that Congress passed the Nursing Home Reform Amendment as part of the Omnibus Budget Reconciliation Act of 1987 to address the issue.[41] A review of psychotropic prescribing practices for nursing home residents suggests that while there has been a decrease in the prescribing of antipsychotic medications since the implementation of the amendment, prescriptions for antidepressants and anxiolytic drugs for this population have increased.[42] Overall, rates of psychotropic drug use in nursing homes have doubled since the 1990s, especially in facilities where doctor–patient contact is minimal.[43] One comprehensive study of more than 12,500 nursing homes between 1996 and 2006 documented a doubling in the proportion of residents receiving psychotropic prescriptions: from 21.9 percent in 1996 to 47.5 percent in 2006.[44] Amazingly, one study found that more than half of new nursing home residents were prescribed psychotropics within two weeks of their admission.[45] The results of polypharmacy can be especially dangerous for elders. Seniors taking nine or more different medications are 2.33 times more likely those taking fewer medications to experience adverse health outcomes, such as hip fractures.[46] Nursing home residents who are subjected to polypharmacy experience more adverse drug events and negative drug-to-drug interactions, lengthier hospitalizations, and higher health care costs.[47] Pharmacoepidemiological studies show that the numbers of psychotropic prescriptions written for nursing home residents are much higher than would seem to be indicated by the reported rates of mental illness in nursing home populations, which suggests rampant overprescribing.

Exactly why nursing home residents are given these drugs is a major issue. Estimates of serious mental illness among nursing home residents vary widely across the United States. In their 2009 study of this topic, Ann Bagchi and her colleagues found that the most reliable estimates were provided by the National Nursing Home Survey, which estimated that only about 6.8 percent of nursing home residents were living with a mental illness.[48] However, other studies have found much higher rates of mental illness in this population. In a study published in 2011, Victor Molinari and colleagues found that 73 percent of elderly nursing home residents had a psychiatric diagnosis at admission, and 85 percent had a psychiatric diagnosis three months after admission.[49] Similarly, Donald Hoover and his colleagues found that 54 percent of nursing home residents received a new diagnosis of depression within the first year of being admitted to the facility: 32 percent were diagnosed at admission, and an additional 21 percent were diagnosed later during the first year.[50]

The fact that psychiatric evaluations are taking place is a good thing, but these assessments often do not seem to matter as much as they should. Many seniors are receiving psychotropics without any appropriate diagnosis of mental illness. It is estimated that between 11 percent and 25 percent of nursing home residents are receiving psychotropic drugs despite a lack of evidence of mental illness.[51] A 2011 audit of seventy-three individual nursing home patient records revealed that while only 73 percent of the residents had a mental health diagnosis at admission, 85 percent were on psychotropics, and 19 percent were on four or more drugs simultaneously. Further, only 50 percent of the residents' files recommended behavioral strategies for coping with forms of distress.[52]

Often, psychotropics are distributed to elders differentially along axes of gender and race. White women younger than eighty-five years of age are more likely than nursing home residents in other groups to receive psychotropics for mental illness, while male residents, non-Hispanic blacks, those eighty-five and older, and residents with severe cognitive and physical impairments are often not appropriately diagnosed and treated for mental illnesses such as depression.[53] Additionally, long-term care facilities that have higher proportions of residents with low levels of education and low socioeconomic status are less likely to give residents the appropriate medications for depression.[54] Elder veterans may be at increased risk of misuse of psychotropic medications; Joseph Hanlon and his colleagues found that nearly 43 percent of elderly veterans were prescribed antidepressants despite having no diagnosed mental illness.[55]

What all of these numbers mean is pretty straightforward. Nursing homes do not need to secure diagnoses of mental illness to prescribe psychotropic drugs to their residents. Drugs that are prescribed in the absence of diagnoses are not intended exclusively to treat legitimate mental health problems—they are intended to make managing the residential home as easy as possible for the staff and as profitable as possible for the facility owners. Keep the beds full, keep the residents quiet. Their actual health and well-being are secondary. The cynicism of this interpretation is supported by the data on elders with dementia, who were the focus of the congressional reforms of the 1980s and the recent Human Rights Watch investigation mentioned earlier.

Increasingly, atypical antipsychotic medications are being prescribed to elderly patients in nursing homes for off-label uses, despite increased risk of stroke, neurological problems, and death.[56] In a study published in 2005, Becky Briesacher and her colleagues found that only 41.8 percent of nursing home residents receiving antipsychotic therapy were being given the drugs in accordance with prescribing guidelines.[57] This kind of drugging results in part from aggressive promotion by pharmaceutical companies. In fact, the largest corporate fraud settlement in U.S. history was the result of a lawsuit over this very issue. Janssen Pharmaceuticals, a Johnson & Johnson subsidiary, was forced to pay $2.2 billion for criminal and civil liability for promoting the off-label use of Risperdal for the treatment of dementia.[58] Nursing homes are the settings for the elder zombie apocalypse.

WARDS OF THE STATE

The third and final institutional crisis that psychotropics are deployed to pacify is the youth foster system, in which, across the United States, nearly 400,000 children are held as wards of the state. Figures reported in 2013 for FY 2012 showed foster children as evenly split between boys and girls, with an average age of nine; 42 percent of them were white, 26 percent were black, 21 percent were Hispanic, and the remaining 11 percent were racial/ethnic "others." In their most recent placements, 47 percent of these children lived with nonrelative foster families, 28 percent with relative foster families, 6 percent in group homes, and 4 percent in preadoptive homes; the remaining 15 percent lived in various situations, including institutions. The average length of time a child spent as a ward of the state was 22.7 months, with just over half of all individuals exiting the system by means of reunification with parents or legal guardians.[59]

The vast majority of children in foster care have already suffered horrific forms of physical and sexual abuse, and many continue to face the threat of death while under state protection. In this context of separation and trauma, psychotropics are ostensibly prescribed to lessen the children's suffering and nurture them back to a state of wellness and wholeness.[60] Rates of psychotropic use in foster care settings are upward of ten times higher than the rates found in community-based samples.[61] Somewhere between 15 percent and 70 percent of children in foster care are drugged, and prescriptions for individuals in this population have been increasing over time across the United States.[62] Indeed, evidence from statewide samples of fostered youth shows that anywhere from 13 percent to 41 percent are prescribed more than one psychotropic at the same time.[63] Across the nation, children living under the auspices of child welfare and protective custody are anywhere from two to four times more likely than children living outside the system to be taking psychotropic drugs. While there is wide variation in practices across the states, in the country as a whole, a study published in 2012 found that 11.8 percent of Medicaid-enrolled youth in the foster care system were using a second-generation antipsychotic, and 5.3 percent were taking a combination of three or more psychotropics.[64]

Researchers have also found gender, racial, and age differences in psychotropic drug use among those in foster care. Several studies have shown that boys are more likely than girls to be prescribed these medications.[65] A 2013 analysis of Medicaid claims in a Mid-Atlantic state found that black youth were more likely than their white counterparts to use psychotropics.[66] At the national level, foster youth ages twelve to sixteen were found to be seven times more likely to use psychotropics than those ages two to five, but the rates for psychotropic use at these young ages are not zero.[67] Differences have also been noted between foster youth living with families and those living in group homes. For example, drawing on a statewide sample of youth in North Carolina, Alfiee Breland-Noble and her colleagues found that those in group homes were 1.8 times more likely to take psychotropics than were those living in foster homes with families.[68] Finally, there is also evidence that the use of psychotropics continues among foster youth even as they "age out" of the system. Ramesh Raghavan and J. Curtis McMillen found that in one state, 13 percent of kids leaving the foster system were still taking at least one psychotropic.[69]

Scholars and mental health practitioners alike have begun to call into question the ethics, inequity, and practicality of current prescribing practices.[70] In fact, some researchers have shown that certain populations who meet the criteria for diagnoses that actually call for the use of psychotropic medications fail to receive adequate treatment.[71] For a study published in 2007, McMillen and his colleagues interviewed 130 child welfare workers and found that they had real concerns about the children in their charge regarding overuse of psychotropic medications, short inpatient stays, and discontinuities in mental health treatment.[72] Some critics have also noted the rising rates of prescribing of psychotropics, which have seen as much as a threefold increase in a ten-year period.[73]

Another point of controversy is the impact that these prescribing practices have on the broader society. Given that the health care of foster youth in the United States is more often than not funded by Medicaid, some scholars have noted the expense to taxpayers represented by the high rates of psychotropic consumption.[74] There is also concern regarding who should be held responsible for these practices; some critics place the responsibility on state and federal agencies, asserting that their lack of oversight in prescribing practices violates international laws intended to protect the welfare of children.[75] Jeffrey Longhofer and his colleagues have argued that the complex nature of the foster system further complicates attempts at collaboration among state, local, and federal agencies on oversight of psychotropic prescribing and use.[76] John Lyons and Laura Rogers question whether children with complicated mental health issues should be in foster care to begin with; perhaps instead they should be placed in other kinds of environments that can better meet their needs, such as inpatient centers.[77]

The scientific and policy debates regarding the use of psychotropic drugging within the custodial institutions discussed in this chapter have unfolded in relative isolation from one another. But these institutions are all in crisis, and they are all linked together. Consider the following connections. Parental deployment as part of military service, parental imprisonment, and serious mental illnesses all contribute to the numbers of children who end up in the child welfare system and foster care.[78] An alarming number of recently returned military veterans find themselves involved with the criminal justice system, as do many adults who, as kids, spent time in the child welfare system.[79] Following deinstitutionalization, nursing homes quickly became primary receptacles for formerly hospitalized mentally ill people and then rapidly expanded due to the fact that Medicaid financed much of these residents' care.[80] Beginning in the 1970s and continuing to the present, direct links can be traced from psychiatric hospital closures to lack of adequate inpatient treatment options to increases in the proportions of jail and prison populations with mental illness.[81] In addition, large numbers of mentally ill people did not flow to other total institutions—they began lives as America's new homeless.[82]

The prisoner who sits warehoused in an overcrowded and overlooked system of mass incarceration, the active-duty soldier who awaits death or disability, the abandoned elder who fears becoming a zombie in a nursing home, the forsaken "problem" child in a group home—all live within the state of psychic emergency made possible by a social structure and culture that cannot recognize, cope with, or substantively remedy their suffering. The meaning of their institutionalization lies at the boundary of their suffering and their mistreatment at the hands of the custodial institutions in which they are held.

We have to interpret this meaning at the boundary of biopolitics and necropolitics. Whether we determine that drugging people en masse is legitimate because it reduces psychic suffering or, conversely, we understand it as illegitimate because it accelerates death by pacifying institutional crisis is contingent on the political logic that justifies the enactment of the practice itself. I do not think that the mass distribution of psychotropic drugs inside custodial institutions is somehow wholly distinct from the broader patterns in so-called free society; rates of psychotropic drug use outside these institutions have also increased dramatically over the past fifty years.[83] Are these drugs therapeutic agents that are supposed to help traumatized people, or are they agents of pacification whose purpose is to quiet already traumatized people? In some ways, it doesn't really matter. In the psychic state of emergency, nearly anything goes. Unless we mobilize to end endless wars, provide substantive care and support for our elders, and provide wraparound platinum care for our young people, the government will continue to use psychotropics to try to keep the peace.

FIVE

THERE ARE DARK DAYS AHEAD

A New Era of Psychic Violence

In February 1974, Dr. Norman Carlson, then the director of the Federal Bureau of Prisons, testified before the House of Representatives Subcommittee on Courts, Civil Liberties, and the Administration of Justice, part of the House Judiciary Committee, at a hearing on behavioral modification programs in the federal prison system. The term *behavioral modification,* as Carlson testified, should be understood as a general and fairly noncontroversial approach to the basic work that correctional institutions do. "In its broadest sense," he argued, "virtually every program in the Bureau of Prisons is designed to change or modify behavior."[1] Carlson was called before the committee to testify about several prison-based behavioral modification programs that had come under intense public scrutiny in the early 1970s: the START program, CARE, and Asklepieion. These programs were the descendants of MKUltra, a secret program of the Central Intelligence Agency that operated from 1953 to 1973 and used psychotropic drugs to extract information from suspects and detainees. The CIA intended to use psychotropics during the Cold War as weapons that would help to secure the new postwar U.S. hegemony. While many drugs in the current crop of psychotropics (SSRIs, second-generation antipsychotics, and powerful tranquilizers) bear little chemical resemblance to the Thorazine and LSD of that period, the new psychotropic weapons have similar politically useful effects, chemically inducing sedation and weakening psychic resistance to legitimate power.

Behavioral modification programs like these are part of a long history of U.S. government efforts to control and change human thoughts and behavior through the application of science, technology, and medicine. The programs used in prisons, which disproportionately targeted

African American, Indigenous, and Latinx inmates, loosely applied techniques in experimental psychology and learning theory to try to reduce violence among prisoners and enforce their compliance with institutional rules. These programs came under fire in the 1970s from critics who argued that they amounted to poorly designed and unethical experiments that enacted unnecessary psychic violence on prisoners.

In his concluding remarks at the congressional hearing, Carlson quoted a few lines from an obscure book on operant conditioning, a specific technique used to change behavior through positive and negative reinforcement, to signal the federal approach not only to behavioral modification but also to the concealment of knowledge about the practice:

> If an organization cooperates with evaluative or monitoring systems, and utilizes novel or experimental techniques, it exposes itself to criticism or possible extinction. . . . On the other hand, if an organization utilizes established noncontroversial methods, and if it conceals—either by commission or omission—its failures or limitations, it is less likely to be criticized and, hence, more likely to survive. It will also be less likely to solve the problem.[2]

What Carlson meant to convey was this: If the Federal Bureau of Prisons wants to experiment with new ways to change behavior, it should do so openly even though its actions are likely to be criticized. If the bureau instead chooses to try the same old ineffective approaches, but does so secretly, it will be subject to less public scrutiny, but the old approaches will not work. From the perspective of the government, the lesson is that it should be bold, experimental, and completely open in its efforts to change people's thoughts and behaviors.

Much as it did during the 1970s with behavioral modification programs in prisons, today the government uses psychotropics to change the thoughts and behaviors of particular groups of people in ways that fall completely outside the boundaries of what is reasonable, ethical, or even medical. Psychotropics are weaponized, used to wage new modes of warfare on criminal, racialized, and sexual enemies of the state.[3] Psychotropics have become indispensable to U.S. national security practices related to international militarized war, border enforcement, and the control of sex crime; they also play an important role in enabling gun violence. I bring these contexts together to document the psychic violence caused by psychotropics that takes place outside the law and in the shadows where science and knowledge cannot penetrate. The government uses psychotropics to wage open psychic war on people it considers to be unruly, dangerous, and illegitimate. And when people use psychotropics, their violence against other people takes on new cultural and political relevance. We should interpret this warfare as necropolitical, a view that frames psychotropics as potent new neurochemical weapons that are used to produce new forms of death. These are institutional uses of psychotropic drugs that extend beyond the borders of therapeutic medicine and beyond custodial institutions that are nominally focused on care, such as those discussed in the previous chapter.

THE "PREFLIGHT COCKTAIL" FOR DETAINED IMMIGRANTS

Clonazepam, divalproex, duloxetine, guanfacine, lurasidone, ziprasidone, olanzapine, clonidine, escitalopram, quetiapine, aripiprazole, chlorpromazine, desmopressin, lamotrigine, lithium, and trazodone—these sixteen drugs were administered to unaccompanied immigrant children held captive at the Shiloh Treatment Center in Manvel, Texas, in 2018 as the result of the Trump administration's policy of separating immigrant families crossing into the United States from Mexico. In April of that year, a memorandum was filed in the U.S. District Court for the Central District of California–Western Division alleging that government workers acting under the aegis the Office of Refugee Resettlement (ORR) had forcibly administered psychotropic drugs to these kids without any demonstration of medical need and without following clearly established rules about their parents' rights to make decisions about their children's health care.[4] The memo further alleged that ORR workers had faked consent forms granting them the power to force the children to take the drugs and had threatened that the children would not be released or would lose access to facility privileges if they did not take the drugs. Noting the extraordinary risk of harm that the use of psychotropic drugs posed for the children, as well as the potential use of such drugs as "chemical straitjackets," the plaintiffs in the case claimed that the ORR preferred autocracy to due process.

While the Trump administration stirred public outrage with its policy of separating immigrant children from their parents, placing them in what were effectively internment camps, and drugging them, it is not widely known that for years, contrary to the agency's own rules and regulations, U.S. Immigration and Customs Enforcement has been forcibly administering psychotropics to civil detainees awaiting trial

and deportation for immigration violations. ICE conservatively estimates that 15 percent of its detainees at any given time suffer from mental illness.[5] Abysmal mental health treatment in immigration facilities
has led to preventable suicides, misdiagnoses, over- and undermedica-
tion, and many lawsuits. While they are obviously important, those detainees judged by ICE to have mental illnesses should not be our only
focus. As in the other institutions I have examined in this book, the
policies that ICE employs ostensibly to facilitate mental health care are
more often used to enable the agency to engage in the infliction of psychic trauma.

From 1940 to 2003, the Immigration and Naturalization Service (INS)
was responsible for implementing federal immigration laws and regulations. Under the purview of INS, the administration of psychotropics
was constricted and conservative. An internal memo issued in November 2000 by Laura Odwazny, an attorney for the U.S. Department of
Health and Human Services during the Clinton administration, sum-
marized this position on chemical restraints.[6] Although civil detainees
are transported on commercial airlines, Odwazny's review of existing
case law found that non-court-ordered involuntary medication of detainees before transport raised ethical concerns and had absolutely no
legal support. INS deemed it appropriate to inject an immigrant detainee with powerful psychotropic medications only when that person
had a mental illness diagnosis and the administration of the drug was
deemed medically necessary.

In 2003, when ICE took over INS functions under the Department
of Homeland Security, it reversed this policy on psychotropics and
permitted the sedation of civil detainees at will. A May 2003 internal
memo from Director Anthony S. Tangeman of ICE's Office of Detention
and Removal clarified the new practice: medical escorts may sedate
an ICE detainee with psychotropics during transport whether or not
the detainee has a diagnosed psychiatric condition if he or she displays
behavior viewed as combative or as threatening to keep ICE from ac-
complishing its mission.[7] Tangeman did not specify what constitutes
combative or threatening behavior.

The Aviation Medicine unit of the Division of Immigration Health
Services, ICE's medical authority, routinely uses high doses of a "preflight cocktail" of Haldol, Ativan, and Cogentin as "chemical restraints"
to facilitate the expatriation of what the government calls combative detainees. ICE has rewritten its rules to allow the use of psychotropics in

"behavioral" contexts in addition to "therapeutic" or psychiatric contexts. Reporting by Amy Goldstein and Dana Priest of the *Washington Post* in 2008 identified more than 250 cases in which detainees were given psychotropics prior to or during deportation, 57 of which involved forced drugging for no apparent medical reason.[8] In 2007, then chief of ICE Julie Myers admitted that 1,073 deportations had taken place between 2003 and 2007 that involved medical escorts from Aviation Medicine.[9]

Yousif Nageib represents one such case. The in-transit medical notes for Nageib's deportation from Dallas, Texas, to the Sudan in January 2007 indicate that he had a "behavioral" medical problem, although the medical escort documented that Nageib was cooperative at the time. ICE agents informed Nageib that there were going to sedate him medically because of previous claims that he "would not go quietly." Although Nageib informed the agents that he would in fact "go quietly" and that he "never said anything" like that, the agents maintained the need to sedate the already calm Nageib with a cocktail of lorazepam, haloperidol, and benzatropine (5–10 milligrams) at doses much higher than recommended for even on-label uses (3–5 milligrams for adults with severe and chronic psychosis).[10]

The potential health consequences of high doses of psychotropics are severe. In September 2007 the U.S. Food and Drug Administration issued an alert concerning intravenous administration of Haldol in high doses, noting increased risk of sudden death even without the presence of predisposing factors such as cardiac abnormalities, hypothyroidism, and familial history of long QT syndrome, a condition that causes fast or irregular heartbeats.[11] As reported by Nina Bernstein in the *New York Times,* ICE has a history of covering up its role in the deaths of detainees in ICE custody, many of whom have gone "uncounted and unnamed."[12] Bernstein documented at least 107 deaths between 2003 and 2008—approximately one every seventeen days. It is unknown how many of these deaths were the result of complications from the forced administration of psychotropics.

In 2007, the American Civil Liberties Union represented Raymond Soeoth and Amadou Diouf in a class action lawsuit against ICE for repeated forced drugging. Both men, in preparation for their deportations (to Indonesia and Senegal, respectively), were forcibly injected with a preflight cocktail. Neither man had any history of mental illness. Soeoth physically resisted officers when they came to take him from his cell, but he gave in to their demands when he saw the needle. He was injected anyway. Diouf was forcibly injected when, while aboard a plane and awaiting takeoff, he insisted that ICE officers allow him to show the pilot a stay of deportation. In January 2008, a civil court found in the two men's favor and awarded Diouf $50,000 and Soeoth $5,000.[13]

There is nothing remotely therapeutic or medical about ICE's use of psychotropics to facilitate the capture and deportation of foreign nationals. The government's standard policy reserving ICE's right to administer psychotropics in behavioral situations is effectively a license for agents to drug people for any reason. In documenting altercations with detainees, agents can always lie about the reasons they administer drugs, if they mention the drugging at all. In the years since the *Washington Post*'s exposé, I have found little public information about these practices, even during the period that President Obama hailed as being an era of open government. Under the aegis of border security and enforcement, ICE deploys whatever weapons it has at its disposal. Under Trump, we are unlikely to hear much at all about this, or about the human beings subjected to forced drugging.

PSYCHIC TORTURE IN THE SO-CALLED WAR ON TERROR

The U.S. Department of Defense has admitted to forcibly administering psychotropics to foreign national detainees in war-zone prisons in Iraq and Afghanistan, at Guantánamo Bay, and within CIA-run "black sites." Such drugging is used prior to so-called extraordinary rendition and during marathon interrogation sessions; psychotropics also function as "chemical restraints," used to manage threatening detainees. Under an operation named Project Medication, the CIA considered using Versed (midazolam), a sedative, as a "truth serum" to aid in extracting intelligence from detainees.[14] We only know about Project Medication because the ACLU sued the federal government to release a report on the operation authored by an unknown agent in the CIA's Office of Medical Services.[15] While the CIA claims that Project Medication never got off the ground due to potential legal objections within the Department of Justice, that is only part of the story.

In 2001, Adnan Latif was arrested at the Pakistan–Afghanistan border because he was suspected of having ties to al-Qaeda. Decades earlier, Latif had suffered a brain injury, and he claimed he was returning from a doctor visit. In 2002, he was sent to the U.S. military detention camp at Guantánamo Bay, Cuba. Over the next eleven years he regularly complained to his lawyer that he was being forced to take drugs that made him feel "like a zombie." In 2012, he ingested two dozen doses of the atypical antipsychotic drug Invega (paliperidone), which he had secretly collected, ending his life. The toxicology report showed a host of painkillers and psychotropics in his system, many of which had dangerous interactions when taken together.[16]

During the time when Latif arrived at Guantánamo it was standard procedure for every arriving detainee to be administered the antimalaria drug mefloquine. The drug was administered not at the preventive dose of 250 milligrams, but at the dose recommended for someone who had already contracted the disease, 1,250 milligrams, despite the government's recognition that malaria was not a threat in Cuba. Mefloquine, especially at the higher dose, can have severe side effects, including vertigo, anxiety, paranoia, hallucinations, depression, psychosis, and suicide. The side effects are the results of changes in brain chemistry caused by the drug and can last long after treatment is discontinued. Mefloquine is one of a group of drugs that the CIA experimented with in the 1950s to induce psychosis as an aid to interrogation.[17] All detainees who arrived at Guantánamo between 2003 and 2007—approximately 249 people—received injections of Mefloquine. Reporting and court documents confirm the use of psychotropics as chemical restraints to subdue terrorism suspects so that they can be transported from one location to another, and as aids to coerce confessions. A 2003 Department of Justice memo, written by the now infamous John Yoo, openly condoned the use of psychotropics on detainees. Yet international law on this subject is clear: the use of psychotropics as so-called truth serum constitutes torture.[18]

Psychotropics are often used as part of a larger interrogation strategy, such as in the case of Abu Zubaydah (given name Zayn al-Abidin Muhammad Husayn), who was captured in 2002 in Pakistan and held at the CIA black site known as Strawberry Fields in Cuba.[19] In addition to receiving Haldol injections, Zubaydah was subjected to at least eighty-three instances of waterboarding and other coercive techniques.[20] Joseph Margulies, attorney for Zubaydah, filed a memo in U.S. district court indicating that when he spoke with Zubaydah, he "felt [he] was talking to an elderly infirm patient whose mind was beginning to fail him."[21] In addition, in the time since Zubaydah had arrived at Guantánamo, he had suffered 116 seizures. Margulies, now professor of law and government at Cornell University, was counsel on the landmark *Rasul v. Bush* (2004) case, in which the U.S. Supreme Court ruled that foreign nationals detained at Guantánamo could file habeas corpus petitions to review whether their detainments were legal.[22] However, in terms of psychotropic use, most federal concern over forced drugging appears to center on whether the drugs were used as part of interrogation strategies.

The reporting on detainees' accusations and on John Yoo's memo in a 2008 *Washington Post* article led Senators Joe Biden (chair of the Senate Foreign Relations Committee), Carl Levin (member of the Senate Armed Services Committee), and Chuck Hagel (senior member of the Senate Select Intelligence Committee and the Senate Foreign Relations Committee) to launch an investigation into allegations of the abuse of detainees with the CIA's Office of the Inspector General.[23] Notably, the investigation found that while the CIA failed to request a legal opinion regarding the use of "mind-altering drugs to enhance interrogations," there was no documented evidence of psychotropic drugging for the purposes of interrogation. However, medical ethicist Leonard Rubenstein of the Johns Hopkins Center for Public Health and Human Rights, who reviewed declassified documents obtained in 2015 by Vice News, told a Vice News reporter that he believed the documents suggested that the "CIA inspector general never conducted a proper investigation, apparently failing to review protocols, medical charts, or interviewed doctors." Whether or not this is true, the CIA certainly entertained the idea. According to Vice News, in 2003 the CIA sponsored a conference that included a session devoted to the question "What pharmacological agents are known to affect apparent truth-telling behavior?"[24]

Functioning as part of a prison system embedded within the military, psychotropics play a role in the War on Terror that is characterized by secrecy, so that the full scope of that role is unknown. In chapter 4, I described how the U.S. military uses psychotropics on active-duty soldiers who are fighting in this war. Here, I have speculated on the little we know about how these drugs are used in coercive interrogations and as chemical restraints on the other side of this amorphous conflict. Psychotropics are not used only against external enemies of the state, however; internal "enemies" such as sex offenders are also subjected to psychotropic drugging.

PSYCHOTROPIC CALMATIVES AND SEXUAL DEATH
IN SEX OFFENDERS

State officials are increasingly administering selective serotonin re-uptake inhibitors to convicted sex offenders as "calmatives" to reduce libido, sexual arousal, sexual fantasy, and the desire to ejaculate. SSRIs, which include Prozac and Lexapro, are antidepressants that increase levels of serotonin in the brain. The state's use of biomedical practices to manage the sexuality of populations first emerged during the early twentieth century with the practices of surgical castration and sterilization—male sex offenders have long been castrated under "eye for an eye" practices.[25] The state's right to sterilize citizens was upheld by the U.S. Supreme Court in *Buck v. Bell* (1927)—in this case a pregnant white woman, Carrie Buck, who had been institutionalized in the Virginia State Colony for Epileptics and Feebleminded after being raped by her adoptive mother's nephew. In the court's decision, Justice Oliver Wendell Holmes Jr. infamously stated, "It is better for all the world, if instead of waiting to execute degenerate offspring for crime . . . society can prevent those who are manifestly unfit from continuing their kind."[26] Carrie Buck's birth mother, who was considered to have a low mental age, had a criminal record of prostitution.

The use of hormonal chemical castration to control violent and aggressive sexuality was first practiced by Dr. Robert Foote in 1944; Foote used diethylstilbestrol, a form of the hormone progesterone (which is involved in menstruation and pregnancy) to manage psychopathy and excessive sex drives in men.[27] During the 1960s German physicians used antiandrogens to constrain male paraphiliacs, and in 1966 the controversial figure Dr. John Money used the hormonal medication medroxy-progesterone acetate (MPA) to reduce abnormal levels of sex drive and sexual fantasies in male sex offenders.[28] The first patient to receive MPA therapy, a twenty-five-year-old man, had sought Money's help regarding his history of cross-dressing.[29] The Upjohn Company manufactures MPA under the trade name Depo-Provera. In women Depo-Provera is approved for use as a contraceptive; in men, the drug decreases testosterone production in the testes and increases testosterone metabolism in the liver. Although Depo-Provera is not FDA approved for use as a treatment for sex offenders, its use in that capacity rose in popularity as studies began to show that recidivism rates remained low among sex offenders receiving this treatment.

In 1969, Alessandro Tagliamonte and colleagues published an article in *Science* describing how rats injected with the serotonin-lowering compound para-chlorophenylalanine became sexually aroused. In contrast, when the rats were given a snack mixed with serotonin, their arousal dissipated.[30] The research, which has been replicated in animal studies, has led psychiatrists to understand sexual deviance through the "monoamine hypothesis," in which monoamines such as dopamine, norepinephrine, and, notably, serotonin drive problematic sexual desires.[31] Within this framework sexual deviance is biologized as serotonin deviance.[32] SSRIs are next-generation antidepressants that increase levels of serotonin in the brain. While the recognized therapeutic uses of SSRIs are the treatment of depression, obsessive-compulsive disorder, and bulimia nervosa, the government recognizes the "off-label" or latent effects of these psychotropics as reducing libido, sexual arousal, sexual fantasy, and ejaculation.[33]

Beginning in the 1990s, soon after the libido-reducing effects of SSRIs were identified, the use of SSRIs such as Prozac, Luvox, Zoloft, and Paxil was introduced as a viable intervention aimed at producing the sexual death of sex offenders.[34] Notably, these drugs have also been suggested for use in nursing home patients with dementia who engage in sexually problematic behavior.[35] In some states, like California, treatment with SSRIs is now a condition of parole for some offenders. In 1996, California became the first state to require certain sex offenders—those who had offended against minors under the age of thirteen at least twice—to submit to weekly Depo-Provera treatments. While California's law is by far the most sweeping of its kind, no legislation involving "chemical castration" that has been enacted thus far in the United States clearly defines that term. This leaves much room for interpretation at the state level regarding which pharmacological treatments achieve "castration."

In a 2009 North American survey, Robert McGrath and his colleagues found that SSRIs were the medications most commonly used to control sexual arousal in sex offenders: these drugs were prescribed for 50.3 percent of offenders in community treatment programs and 55.3 percent of offenders in residential treatment programs.[36] Psychiatrists have suggested that SSRIs are appropriate for use with "low-risk" offenders, identified as those who are self-referred, those who are open about their offenses, those who have offended against known (rather than stranger) victims, those who have committed hands-off offenses, first-time offenders, and offenders with nonparaphilic preference.[37] Few clinical trials have been conducted to evaluate the effectiveness of SSRI therapy for sex offenders, but the use of SSRIs is often viewed as preferable to traditional chemical castration, by both psychiatrists and offenders, because SSRIs have fewer perceived side effects than Depo-Provera and the cost of SSRIs is lower.[38] However, it is likely that SSRIs are preferable from another angle—they offer a way to "avoid throwing the baby out with the bathwater." Dr. Martin Kafka, a psychiatrist, has suggested that SSRIs can dampen deviant sexual urges while amplifying normative sexual urges.[39] In order to achieve this goal with greater precision, John Bradford created an algorithm for treatment based on the effects of various drugs and the six treatment levels for the four categories of paraphilia described in the *Diagnostic and Statistical Manual of Mental Disorders* (third edition, revised).[40] In 2016, the World Federation of Societies of Biological Psychiatry (formed in 1974), which provides guidance to institutions on psychiatry-related protocols, proposed an updated version of Bradford's SSRI algorithm.[41]

The question of how to reduce reoffending by those who commit sexual violence is one of the government's most intractable criminological problems. The ethics of administering psychotropics to convicted sex offenders are always fraught, yet this practice seems like an updated technoscientific version of "eye for an eye" retribution. Requiring offenders to subject themselves to this dystopian version of neurochemical castration seems to violate basic human rights, even if it is permitted by U.S. law. Whether these drugging practices actually reduce instances of sexual violence is unknown. In addition to seeking answers to that question, perhaps we should also ask whether psychotropics increase the likelihood of people committing gun violence.

DO PILLS MAKE PEOPLE USE GUNS TO KILL PEOPLE?
A CASE STUDY OF GEORGE ZIMMERMAN

The role that psychotropics might play in enabling violence has taken on new national significance in the context of the ongoing epidemic of gun violence and mass shootings in the United States. The perpetrators' names and the locations of their horrific crimes are now etched into the American national consciousness: Eric Harris and Dylan Klebold in Columbine, James Holmes in Aurora, Adam Lanza in Newtown, Nidal Hasan at Fort Hood, Cho Seung-Hui at Virginia Tech. These tragedies are always followed by debates about access to mental health care and the role that psychotropics may have played in pushing the perpetrators into violent behavior. There is a disturbing body of medical literature that connects the use of psychotropics to aggressive and violent behavior. Even when they have been prescribed and used in ways consistent with sound psychiatric practice, psychotropic medications have been associated with suicide, homicide, and other forms of interpersonal violence.[42] When overused and abused, evidence suggests, psychotropics can literally be deadly, both for the users and for those with whom they come in contact.

On February 27, 2012, the morning after he shot and killed seventeen-year-old Trayvon Martin in Sanford, Florida, George Zimmerman was examined by Lindzee E. Folgate, the attending physician assistant at the Altamonte Family Practice.[43] Described in the medical record as a twenty-eight-year-old white male, Zimmerman told this health care provider that he was taking several psychotropic medications—Restoril, Adderall, and Librax.[44] Restoril is a brand name for temazepam, which is a benzodiazepine tranquilizer, one of a subclass of psychotropics that are commonly used to treat insomnia and have been associated with physical and gun violence and getting into trouble with police, especially when paired with alcohol consumption.[45] In 1996, the British government reclassified temazepam as a Schedule 3 drug (making possession of it without a prescription illegal) after it was associated with numerous serious violent events and deaths among British youth.[46] In the mid-1990s, Restoril was the most widely abused prescription drug in Great Britain. In 2007, the FDA imposed stricter labeling requirements on drugs like Restoril because they had been found to be associated with an increase in dangerous sleep-related behaviors, like "sleep-driving."[47]

Adderall is an amphetamine and stimulant that is used to treat the symptoms associated with attention-deficit/hyperactivity disorder and narcolepsy; the FDA currently requires a black-box warning on Adderall packaging highlighting the drug's addictiveness. MedlinePlus lists among Adderall's serious side effects "feeling unusually suspicious of others," "hallucinations," and "aggressive or hostile behavior."[48] In an aftermarket pharmacoepidemiological analysis of reports of adverse drug events received by the FDA from 2004 through 2009, amphetamine (one of two generic ingredients in Adderall) was found to be related to thirty-one violent events and was 9.6 times more likely to be linked to violence than other drugs in the adverse event reporting system.[49] Librax is a habit-forming combination of chlordiazepoxide and clidinium bromide that is used to treat ulcers and bowel disorders. While Librax is not a psychotropic drug itself, it can have psychological side effects like "aggression," "being easily annoyed" and "losing one's sense of reality or identity."[50] MedlinePlus indicates that stopping Librax suddenly can also create "anxiousness, irritability, and sleeplessness"; Zimmerman's medical records are unclear on whether he was taking Librax consistently.[51] The use of Librax is contraindicated for individuals who are taking benzodiazepines like Restoril, and it should not be combined with alcohol consumption; the combination of Librax, Restoril, and alcohol can exacerbate known side effects, create new side effects, or pose new risks to the user's body.[52]

The Sanford Police Department did not administer any alcohol or drug tests to Zimmerman, either on the night of the shooting or during his subsequent questioning at the station.[53] Two cheek swabs were taken from Zimmerman on the night of the shooting, but they were used only to establish a genetic match with bodily fluids found on other forms of evidence collected at the scene.[54] Had George Zimmerman been drinking the day of the shooting? Did he have other illicit drugs in his body? If he had consumed alcohol that night, he would likely have experienced an adverse and paradoxical reaction to the combination of alcohol with Librax and Restoril that would probably have shaped his mental state. We will never know what substances were circulating in his body that night, but we do know that Zimmerman had an alcohol-related brush with the law back in 2005. He was arrested and charged with felony obstruction of justice and battery against a police officer in Orange County, Florida, for pushing and resisting an officer without violence (a misdemeanor). Further prosecution was waived after Zimmerman entered an alcohol education program.[55]

Zimmerman was tried for the killing of Trayvon Martin, and in July 2013 he was acquitted of second-degree murder and manslaughter. If the jurors had had a clearer picture of Zimmerman's drug use, violent past, and mental health instability, might they have arrived at a different conclusion about his guilt? In addition to his 2005 arrest, Zimmerman had been accused of sexually molesting a female cousin over a period of ten years, and a former fiancée had sought a restraining order against him for domestic violence.[56] In November 2013, not long after his trial for the killing of Martin, Zimmerman was detained on charges of domestic violence for a second time, but the charges were eventually dropped.[57]

Either deliberately or inadvertently, the prosecution in the Trayvon Martin case and the news media downplayed or ignored Zimmerman's history of violence and psychotropic use as a potentially important factor in the case. For reasons that can only be speculated about—such as the possibility that Zimmerman's father, a former Virginia magistrate, intervened on his behalf with the Sanford Police Department to close records related to his multiple arrests—Zimmerman's mental state was not scrutinized, in contrast to the cases of other perpetrators of gun violence.[58] The failure of both prosecution and news media to introduce evidence of Zimmerman's past violent behavior, mental health status, and ongoing use of psychotropic drugs contributed to people seeing Zimmerman's actions against Martin as normal, reasonable, and justified, particularly in a world obsessed with white people's safety and security. The paranoia that Zimmerman expressed about Martin's presence in the Sanford neighborhood during a 911 call was explained away by his defense team as a response to earlier burglaries in the area. But that does not explain why Zimmerman ignored the police dispatcher's statement that it was not necessary for him to follow Martin. It also does not explain why Zimmerman was carrying a gun in the residential community, or why he chose to take the gun with him to follow an unknown teen who was apparently not doing anything illegal.

There are insurmountable evidentiary challenges to proving that psychotropics *caused* Zimmerman to follow and kill Trayvon Martin. It is possible, though highly speculative, that the introduction of expert testimony regarding the known correlation between the consumption of the drugs that Zimmerman was taking and instances of aggression and violence might have changed both the public and the legal discourse about this case. Further, the fact that such discussion has taken place in reference to mass shootings but was conspicuously missing from the analysis of the factors in this case raises the question of why. Despite the fact that Zimmerman's medical records were available to them, the prosecutors never suggested that the consumption of psychotropics may have caused Zimmerman to kill Martin.[59]

The fact that a number of perpetrators of mass shootings have experienced episodes of serious mental illness prior to and at the times of their crimes has become a widely circulated and oversimplified explanation for their violence—suggesting that only the psychically unwell can engage in violence of this magnitude. The presence of mental illness signals the abnormality of the perpetrators themselves, which serves as the de facto cause of their violent behavior. Taking psychotropics, in and of itself, is not generally thought to be a potential causal factor in these violent behaviors. Clearly, most people who use psychotropic drugs do not commit violence, either on themselves or on others. Still, using psychotropics is framed as a medically sanctioned and rational response to mental illness and therefore cannot be framed as causally related to violence itself. Psychotropics are supposed to *prevent* violence, not *enact* or *enable* it, right?

Like so many of the other questions raised in this book, this one poses a difficult empirical problem. It is a real scientific challenge to prove that psychotropics cause people (nearly exclusively men) to commit crimes such as mass shootings, but the observed correlation between the consumption of these drugs and instances of violent crime requires closer empirical scrutiny. Basically, there are two ways in which scientists can analyze the relationship between psychotropics and violent behavior: they can examine reports of violent events and/or thoughts during human clinical trials *before* a drug is approved by the Food and Drug Administration for distribution in the United States, or they can examine reports made back to the FDA about adverse drug reactions that involve violent behaviors and/or thoughts *after* a drug has been released into the market. Strictly speaking, neither analytic strategy can provide ironclad proof that a specific compound or combination of compounds will cause an individual to commit a specific act of violence with or without a gun; such analyses can only document an *association* between a specific drug and an event in any group of people. Moreover, current FDA regulations require that drug manufacturers conduct human clinical trials only on individual drugs, not on drug combinations that people are likely to consume. To complicate this empirical problem further, it is not possible to prove that the consumption of a psychotropic drug caused a specific individual to commit violence independent of other factors that shaped the violent event itself. Therefore, we can only speculate about how psychotropics might be shaping endemic gun violence in the United States.

The correlation between gun violence and serious mental illness has informed national and state policy responses to such violence, including the passage of state laws regulating the sale of firearms to people with mental illness and new proposals to register persons with mental illness for the ostensible purposes of violence prevention.[60] In reality, however, persons with mental illness are more likely to be the victims of violent crime than its perpetrators.[61] A federal statute states that "any person who is an unlawful user of or addicted to marihuana or any depressant, stimulant, or narcotic drug, or any person who has been adjudicated a mental defective or has been committed to any mental institution" cannot receive, transport, dispose of, or possess a firearm in the United States.[62] On February 5, 2016, the Obama administration changed the Health Insurance Portability and Accountability Act of 1996 to give permission to federal mental health care providers to report persons with serious mental illnesses to the National Instant Criminal Background Check System so that they could be identified if they attempted to ship, transport, possess, or receive firearms. Persons subject to this new reporting are

> individuals who have been involuntarily committed to a mental institution; found incompetent to stand trial or not guilty by reason of insanity; or otherwise have been determined by a court, board, commission, or other lawful authority to be a danger to themselves or others or to lack the mental capacity to contract or manage their own affairs, as a result of marked subnormal intelligence or mental illness, incompetency, condition, or disease.[63]

The state of Florida complies with federal law prohibiting the sale of firearms to persons who are "mental defectives," and the state will not provide a permit to carry a concealed weapon to any person who has been

> committed to a mental institution, under Chapter 394 or similar laws of any other state, unless the applicant produces a certificate from a licensed psychiatrist stating that he or she has not suffered from disability for at least five years prior to the date of submission of the application.[64]

The hope is that prevention policies like these can either preemptively identify persons who are likely to engage in violent behavior or reduce the impact of their violence by limiting their access to lethal weapons.

There are dark days ahead. In June 2018, the Minneapolis *Star Tribune* reported that emergency medical services workers for Hennepin County (where Minneapolis is located) had injected criminal suspects with the powerful tranquilizer ketamine, often at the behest of Minneapolis police officers.[65] In some cases, these injections caused severe breathing trouble and even stopped people's hearts, leading to intubations and re-suscitations. The *Star Tribune's* reporting was based on a not-yet-public investigation by the Office of Police Conduct Review, part of the Min-neapolis Department of Civil Rights, which found that EMS workers had injected sixty-two people with ketamine in 2017, up from three in 2012. Current policy permits EMS workers to use chemical sedation if a person is "profoundly agitated," but none of the cases reviewed in the internal investigation seemed to meet that criterion; indeed, some of the people were already handcuffed when they were injected. They were merely criminal suspects.

The patterns of abuse in all of the cases outlined here are strik-ingly similar. Our laws grant institutions the power to administer psy-chotropic drugs to captive populations, even when specific people in those populations do not need or want the drugs, and even when that drugging supports unjust policy choices and social inequality. This government-sanctioned and -funded psychotropic drugging is happen-ing on an unprecedented scale, although it is not always easy to docu-ment exactly what individual institutions are doing to people. When we get a chance to peek through the barbed-wire fences and the blue cur-tains, we have to pay close attention to how our government treats the least among us. Psychotropic drugging may or may not be legal, and it may or may not be based on sound medical evaluation, but we have to ask the bigger question: Is the targeted psychotropic drugging of people in captivity by our government humane?

The answer to this question is no. Such practices weaponize medi-cine for the purposes of carrying out state violence and repression. While U.S. citizens have the right to contest forced drugging in court, the government can forcibly administer psychotropics indefinitely to any person believed to be a threat to him- or herself, to others, or to property. Thus, citizens' constitutional rights to bodily integrity and not to be tortured are positioned against the raw police power of the state to produce safety and security at seemingly any cost. These captive people cannot easily protest government abuses of the power to drug. The surreptitious role that psychotropics play in the government's ef-forts to change people's behavior, whether on the border, on the battle-field, or on the streets, remains shrouded in darkness. This new era of psychic violence features institutional uses of psychotropics that shock the conscience, yet we do not know the full scope and shape of such violence. We know that ICE is using psychotropics on immigrants, but we do not have a complete picture of the penetrations of body and mind committed by this government agency in the name of secure borders. We know that the U.S. military is using psychotropics on what it calls enemy combatants, but we do not know exactly how it is subordinating the flesh of brown men to gain information about the so-called enemy's plans. We know that criminal justice officials are using psychotropics to deaden the sexuality of persons who have been convicted of sexual violence, but at what cost to civil liberty and our purportedly shared humanity? We suspect that psychotropics *have something to do* with the nation's epidemic of gun violence, but we are left to wander in speculation and drown in our suspicions while the bloodshed continues. If the story about psychotropics in American society is as much about death and the creation of suffering as it is about health and the healing of psychic wounds, as this chapter has suggested, how can we begin to move out of the shadows and into the light?

In the current political moment, where blatantly cruel and inhumane immigration policies, unbridled uses of lethal force by police, and summary executions via drone strikes have placed black and brown people within the government's crosshairs, the delicate balance of power that should define an ethical, democratic society has been upended. Given the dangerous combination of racist policy and callous uses of power we have witnessed in the Trump administration's treatment of immigrant children—separating them from their families, holding them in detention camps, and forcibly drugging them—we should expect more dark days ahead.

OVERDOSE

Institutional Addiction in the U.S. Carceral State

Is it possible for the U.S. carceral state to exist without psychotropics? We do not have access to all of the evidence we would need to answer this question directly, at least when it comes to prisons. But if we are thinking about the broader U.S. carceral state, not only the prison–industrial complex and all of its institutional diversity but also all of the other networked custodial institutions that rely heavily on psychotropic drugs— the active-duty military, the foster care system, elder care institutions, ICE—I think we can say the answer is *no*. If we, as a society, were not drugging millions of people living within custodial institutions, there is no way these institutions could continue to function as we currently expect them to. Psychotropic drugging has become business as usual, the accepted protocol, the rule rather than the exception, the go-to therapy, the frontline treatment for a disordered society. We are literally overdosing on psychotropics, and we could not maintain policies of mass captivity without them. My intention in this book has been to document the patterns of institutional abuse involving psychotropics throughout captive America.

We have reached a point where these institutions cannot do what we have given them the power to do if they do not use brain-altering drugs that magically allow them to manage the thoughts and behaviors of human beings. They cannot function without psychotropics. In other words, the institutions that make up the carceral state, some of the most powerful institutions in the United States, are completely hooked— literally addicted to and dependent on these drugs. And this has become a massive, hidden, and taken-for-granted problem in our society because it conceals inhumane practices of confinement that allow us to hold millions of people against their will by directly changing their will. The latest edition of the *Diagnostic and Statistical Manual of Mental Disorders (DSM-5)* frames substance use disorders as involving "a problematic pattern of use of an intoxicating substance leading to clinically significant impairment or distress."[1] If we redefine substance use disorders from the individual level to the level of social institutions, based on the analysis presented in the preceding chapters, we can begin to understand substance abuse as maladaptive patterns of *institutional* substance use leading to *socially* significant impairment or distress.

It may sound metaphorical or hyperbolic to talk about social institutions having human problems, but institutions can be like people in important socially recognized ways. We often use metaphors to talk about social institutions, frequently likening them to human bodies: they can grow or shrink, they can be strong or weak, they can be sick or healthy; they are born, and they can die. We talk about and interact with institutions as if they have bodies, as if they are bodies, as if they can have bodily experiences. And we have long since moved beyond merely metaphorical representations of institutions as bodies to legally inscribed ones. The idea of corporate personhood is one example of this phenomenon. This concept is important because it allows us to see how we can talk about, interact with, and analyze institutions as if they are bodies. The literal meaning of *incorporation* is to form into a body. In the words of the perennial Republican candidate Mitt Romney, "Corporations *are* people, my friend." The term *corporate personhood* refers to the idea that institutions have certain constitutional rights just as persons do—they have private property rights and can enter into contracts, they have the right to free speech, and they have the right to sue in court (to defend said rights). These personal powers, such as the power to make unlimited contributions to political campaigns and the power to defend and advance their interests in U.S. courts, are essential for corporations' engagement in modern forms of capitalist exploitation. Corporate personhood has been affirmed by the U.S. Supreme Court since the passage of the Fourteenth Amendment, perhaps most famously and controversially in the 2010 case *Citizens United v. Federal Election Commission*.[2] If we think about our institutions as persons, as *Citizens United* has us doing, how can we know if our institutional bodies have a drug problem? Let's run through a quick symptom checklist based on some commonsense criteria for identifying substance use disorders: spending a lot of money, losing control over use, developing tolerance, and quitting.

First, like drug addicts, custodial institutions spend lots and lots of money (deep into the multiple billions) on psychotropic drugs, busting their medical budgets to keep the drugs in stock and flowing. Thus, the commodification of captives' mental health services constitutes an important site of overdose. If our institutions are addicted to psychotropics, then who are the drug dealers? The global pharmaceutical industry's financial interests in maintaining the U.S. carceral state's dependence on psychotropics must be confronted head-on. We need to pay closer attention to these financial interests as they intersect with the interests of the prison–industrial complex. As I have argued in this book, prison pharmaceutical regimes encompass networks of institutions, regulations, and technologies that manage the prescribing, procurement, distribution, and disposal of pharmaceuticals. As I have shown in chapter 2, performing a comprehensive and system-wide audit of prison pharmaceutical regimes is a difficult if not impossible task. When we add prisons to the other custodial institutions considered in this book, a picture emerges of the largest system for the procurement and distribution of psychotropic drugs in the world. Every dollar spent by the government for the health of prisoners is a dollar received by a private health corporation—prisons, and the prisoners within them, represent an important node in the circuitry of biocapitalism. The U.S. carceral state, in all of its institutional diversity, is the single largest purchaser of psychotropic drugs in the world by far.

Second, just as drug addicts eventually lose control over their lives, including any semblance of control over when and under what conditions they use, institutions have lost bureaucratic control over how they use psychotropics. As I have documented in chapter 2, prisons experience real difficulties in managing their pharmacy operations, to the point where many seem to have no idea what drugs are coming in, who is getting what, and why. The weakness of mechanisms of administrative oversight and accountability creates a context ripe for abuses. The systematic treatment of elders, youth in the foster system, and soldiers documented in chapter 4 demonstrates this problem. Not knowing when and why a drug is distributed complicates efforts to ensure that people are being treated well and cared for properly. It is just and medically responsible to provide medicines to people who suffer—it is unjust and unconscionable to give medicines to people so that institutions do not suffer.

Third, just as drug addicts experience tolerance, meaning that the physiological effects of the drugs wear off despite increased use, institutions have developed a kind of tolerance, distributing more and more drugs to lesser effect, leading to the use of ever more powerful drugs and drug combinations. The problems of psychotropic polypharmacy in prisons, nursing homes, and the foster system all speak to this symptom of tolerance. As evidenced by how we treat immigrant detainees, sex offenders, and enemy combatants, we are using psychotropics in coercive ways that shock the conscience.

Finally, just as addicts may try to quit but just cannot seem to let the drugs go, institutions have engaged in persistent but unsuccessful efforts to control their use of psychotropics, to the point where they have had to be sued in court or closely regulated before they have been able to check their use. Legislative and policy efforts to curtail the use of psychotropics have had weak and inconsistent effects on patterns of institutional drug use. And like addicts, institutions continue to use drugs despite negative consequences. As discussed in chapter 4, nursing homes offer an instructive case: legislators, regulators, and health professionals have tried for decades to regulate the distribution of psychotropics in these facilities, and their efforts have been only partially and temporarily successful.

U.S. custodial institutions are psychotropic addicts, but simply using drugs to excess, as I have described, does not make one an addict. As is often the case with drug use in individuals, institutional drug use is a *symptom* of a much deeper emotional or affective problem. I believe that affective problem has to do with the structure of psychiatric power in American society, the kind of power that justifies the pacification of captive populations.

CHALLENGING PSYCHIATRIC POWER

To borrow from Dr. Benjamin Rush, a so-called founding father of both American psychiatry and penology, the emergence of the science of psychiatry raised the possibility of governing mad people without the use of chains and whips.[3] For Rush, as for many of psychiatry's early practitioners, there was hope that a medical science of mental illness could transcend the moralizing religious dogmas that had defined the treatment of madness up to that time and help people live better lives. Psychiatry produces a powerful medical narrative to justify psychotropic drug use because psychotropics are most often distributed to captive populations in the name of improving mental health. How does this justification work?

Michel Foucault uses the term *psychiatric power* to describe a way of directing a will in revolt and yoking that will to a new institutionally defined reality—an intensification of reality. According to Foucault, a medical stamp granted the eighteenth-century asylum doctor (a proto-psychiatrist) the power to redirect the will of the captive. This medical stamp was unrelated to what the doctor knew, and it was not justified through any specific scientific knowledge that the doctor used in practice—rather, this medical stamp was conferred as long as the doctor was present in the institution and put five "tokens of knowledge" to work in the asylum.[4] One of these tokens of knowledge was "the double register of medication and direction":

> When a patient has done something that one wants to curb, he must
> be punished, but in punishing him one must make him think that
> that one punishes him because it is therapeutically useful. One must
> therefore be able to make the punishment function as a remedy and,
> conversely, when one fixes a remedy for him, one must be able to
> impose it knowing that it will do him good, but making him think
> that it is only to inconvenience and punish him. This double game
> of remedy and punishment is essential to how the asylum functions
> and can only be established provided that there is someone who
> presents himself as possessing the truth concerning what is remedy
> and what is punishment.[5]

This historical interpretation mirrors what has been said about the use of psychotropic drugs under a policy of technocorrections. The boundary between punishment and therapy is necessarily blurry because it does not rely on or require actual knowledge of mental health—mental health is largely irrelevant to the question of institutional uses of psychotropics. Rather, as Foucault argues, the medical stamp establishes "a game between the mad person's subjected body and the psychiatrist's institutionalized body, the psychiatrist's body extended to the dimensions of an institution."[6] Wherever there were psychiatrists, the medical stamp and its tokens of knowledge justified the subordination of the body and will of the captive. This psychiatric power subsequently migrated out of the eighteenth-century asylum and into a whole set of disciplinary institutions where "it is necessary to make reality function as power."[7]

The last major intellectual movement to challenge the political game of psychiatry was called *antipsychiatry*. This movement, which emerged in the 1950s, had its heyday in the 1960s, and began to wind down in the 1970s, was opposed to legally sanctioned treatment within custodial institutions, challenged the assumptions of biological etiologies of mental illness, critiqued standardized nosology of mental illness, raised concerns about the dehumanizing dynamics of doctor–patient relationships in mainstream psychiatry, and worked to undermine the functions of psychiatry within disciplinary institutions and normalizing societies.[8] Led by psychiatrists and scholars in the United States, England, Italy, and France, the antipsychiatry movement had intellectual roots in the new leftist politics of the period, which were connected to strains of Marxism, libertarianism, and anarchism.

It is important to make a distinction between antipsychiatry as the historically specific intellectual and social movement described above and a broader set of critiques of psychiatry and its frame for mental illness that continues to emerge. These latter critiques of psychiatric power have come from analysts, historians, practitioners, and lay advocates, and they are not all "antipsychiatry." Compared with the earlier movement, the ongoing challenges to psychiatric power involve more voices (rather than only those of a relatively small group of European men), with new questions being asked about such things as the intersection of "mental" disability with social structures like racism, sexism, heterosexism, ageism, and nationality. The antipsychiatrists did not directly question how these axes of domination and resistance shaped the practices within psychiatry with which they were most concerned, nor did they ever consider how social hierarchies influenced their opposition to psychiatry. To their credit, they did often take account of social class. But it would be feminists, critical race theorists, and postcolonial agitators who would raise these issues in their own analyses. If we consider antipsychiatry's essential critiques about institutionalization, diagnostic classification, etiological theory, and treatment regimes, it seems as if people of color, women, queer folks, the young and old, and colonial subjects were especially vulnerable to psychiatric violence. To be made into a subject of psychiatric violence was to enter into the fold of mechanisms of domination that were closely linked to forms of white supremacist capitalist heterosexist patriarchy in both the United States and Europe. We have to remember that psychiatry is a Western social formation that became a politically and economically useful export for these modern forms of governance.

Does antipsychiatry retain any potential to offer criticisms that might be useful in the effort to abolish the U.S. carceral state? Which audiences immediately tune out when they hear the word *antipsychiatry*? Like *socialism* or *abolitionism*, the word comes with unwarranted, pre-fabricated meanings that reduce its rhetorical power. I am confident that people in positions of power are not interested in engaging in conversation with antipsychiatrists. I can see the utility of a strategic re-branding of antipsychiatry that would broaden the bandwidth of those who might listen, those who must listen, those who want to listen. But at what cost would this rebranding come?

In the United States, the dominant psychiatric modalities against which the original antipsychiatrists responded were already in decline by the time antipsychiatry gained visibility. In the early 1960s, the birth of a new discourse of "mental health"—as opposed to the immediately prior discourse of "mental hygiene" that accompanied the political decision to close state psychiatric hospitals—served to deflate the targets of antipsychiatrists' critique. The population high for state psychiatric asylums in the United States came in 1955, *before* the critiques of anti-psychiatrists Thomas Szasz and Erving Goffman, before R. D. Laing and David Cooper. It would be nonsense to argue that they were successful in challenging a process that was already becoming a thing of the past. In fact, it was journalists and other observers, not the antipsychiatrists, who brought the inhumanity of the asylum into public consciousness and spurred state reform efforts. So it seems that the therapeutic state the antipsychiatrists were fighting was already in retreat. Moreover, the more radical premises of their critiques of psychiatry, and of the therapeutic state in which psychiatry increasingly played a role, really only circulated among like-minded leftists and did not have much effect on public understanding or state policy. I doubt that the antipsychiatrists had any lasting or serious impact on national mental health policy in the United States, or on the practice of psychiatry more generally, despite their time in the limelight.

We need to question whether psychiatry is the proper domain in which to ask and answer questions about mental health. Simply questioning the empirical basis of psychiatric disorders does not amount to a negation of their reality in people's lives. Many antipsychiatrists take the view that psychiatric disorders (as articulated in the *DSM-5* and through psychoanalytic theories) are socially and culturally constructed. Many scholars in the field of science and technology studies also take the view that the human sciences and the knowledge produced through them are fundamentally social and cultural in nature. According to these interpretations, there is no true knowledge that exists outside of particular social and cultural contexts. Questioning the objective truth of psychiatric knowledge does not disallow the subjective experience of mental illness, it just means that the scientist's claim to truth is subject to social and cultural analysis and critique. To say it plainly, just because an author says that an illness is socially constructed, that does not mean that it is not experienced. I think we can question knowledge and embrace experience at the same time. How can the insights of antipsychiatry be brought to bear on the future of mental health science and policy in the United States? If you want to reform an institution, you want the people in power at the table with the reformers. But if you want to abolish an institution, certain conversations are immediately off the table when you negotiate and engage in dialogue with power in revolutionary terms. The first thing that is not up for debate is power itself. If, on the contrary, you aim to dismantle psychiatry and the custodial power of the state altogether, you want to burn the table down, or break its legs, or at least steal it and donate it to someone who needs a table. That is what I have tried to accomplish with this book—to break one of the legs on which the U.S. carceral state stands. Without psychotropics, the system cannot stand up.

TOWARD SOBRIETY, TRANSPARENCY, AND PSYCHIC FREEDOM

If our institutions are hooked on drugs, how do we help them sober up and begin a process of recovery? Well, the first step in sobering up is accepting the fact that you have a problem and that the situation is completely out of control. Viewing the issue through a wider sociological lens, we can see that there are many more custodial institutions with psychotropic drug problems that I have not considered in this book. What about kids and schools? What about veterans and the Veterans Administration? What about everyday workers and our completely run-amok version of capitalism? If practices of captivity have extended into the brain, our rulers do not need "chains and whips" to keep other people under control.

To confront these institutional drug problems, we also have to do what twelve-step programs call an "inventory" of psychotropic drug use in institutions. We have to demand much more transparency. Social institutions such as prisons are famously closed off from the rest of society—this closure encompasses not only the people who live and work in the institutions but also the information, the knowledge, about what exactly is going on inside those walls. We struggle to understand what is going on inside the U.S. carceral state. What role does this vast system really play in our society? Should we accept the stated official versions of what is going on, like this one offered by the Federal Bureau of Prisons, "We protect public safety by ensuring that federal offenders serve their sentences of imprisonment in facilities that are safe, humane, cost-efficient, and appropriately secure, and provide reentry programming to ensure their successful return to the community"?[9] Or should we turn to more political interpretations offered by people who are subject to captivity? In these versions, prisons are designed to break people and murder spirits. They are sites for the extraction of political and economic profit from the brains and bodies of people.

This may be the largest, most unscientific natural experiment in the history of biomedicine: What happens when you give large quantities of often powerful mind-altering substances to large-scale human populations? As psychotropic drugging has continued to increase in U.S. society, and indeed around the world, I have been thinking about this grand experiment. I am deeply worried about the results. This is the most dangerous kind of human experiment, the kind where no scientists are collecting and interpreting the data. Until we demand and get full transparency, we will continue to spiral down into the black hole of addiction, loss, and pain.

Another way of framing this conversation about institutional addiction is in terms of our increasing dependence on technologies to solve what are fundamentally social problems. Institutions have always found it useful to employ technologies, including psychotropics, to establish and facilitate subordination. In her masterful book *The New Jim Crow*, Michelle Alexander argues that the U.S. prison system constitutes a new form of structural racism formed largely by the so-called War on Drugs, racist social and economic policies, and the circulation of cultural ideas about racial groups.[10] This new caste system has generated gross forms of political disenfranchisement, social dislocation, and human suffering. Alexander's book shines a new conceptual light on the racist structure and political meaning of mass incarceration, enabling us to see the prison system as a new form of Jim Crow. Yet Alexander's only focus on technology has to do with the militarization of the police, a problem in its own right. Alexander describes the ways in which local and state police forces have become literal armies—stocked with military equipment from the Pentagon and funded by civil forfeiture of citizens' assets and property—that carry out operations on American streets. For example, we continue to see military-style deployments of police forces in response to citizen uprisings against police brutality in African American communities and protests by Native Americans against the desecration of sovereign tribal lands. But might Alexander be missing something really important about the broader role of technologies in creating and maintaining not only the prison system but also the entire U.S. carceral state?

As the prison–industrial complex has grown in political and cultural importance and structural complexity, its overseers have had to develop and deploy new tools to keep it functioning smoothly. As carceral technologies that social actors use to create and reproduce cultures and structures of mass confinement, psychotropic drugs have transformed the ways in which the carceral state is achieved and maintained in the United States. The meaning of *carceral technologies* that I want to embrace here is one that centers how technologies have agency to act in the world.[11] We have to recognize simultaneously both the power of technologies to shape social life and the ways in which technologies themselves operate as forms of power in social life. These are two separate things. People in positions of power use technologies as tools to achieve desired, often potentially unjust, ends. These technologies have become integrated into the functioning of the entire society, not just the U.S. prison system, and themselves require the construction of social systems that make their use seem reasonable, normal, and legitimate. Technologies also have their own agency because they require people in positions of power to build specialized operating environments for their use.[12] I take the position that we must analyze how technologies are used and oppose their use in ways that support the regeneration of unjust social systems including militarism, racism, patriarchy, heterosexism, ableism, capitalism, and colonialism.

Carceral technologies are used in multiple ways to create and sustain the prison–industrial complex and other institutions of mass confinement in the United States, but they have also created a social and political environment in which so-called free citizens are subjected to technological manipulation and pacification. Technologies have world-building agency. We must oppose the use of technologies in unjust ways that require us to build unjust worlds. And technological dependence is a big problem in societies like ours, for two reasons. First, by drugging people en masse, we are simply snipping away at the symptoms of a much deeper social disease—the dynamics of inequality, dislocation, and confrontation that define our society. Second, shortsighted technological fixes invariably generate unanticipated consequences—they become problems in and of themselves. So, what are the unanticipated consequences of technological dependence, of institutional addiction? More important, what can we do about them?

In this book I have aimed, to the fullest extent permissible by available evidence, to dislodge the dominant and partial narrative of psychotropics as agents of healing in favor of a more nuanced view that recognizes these drugs' great potential as instruments of human suffering. Theoretically, we need to shift the study of biotechnologies like psychotropics away from the domain of health and biopolitics and toward an examination of the widespread deployment of these biotechnologies in the context of psychic death and necropolitics. I believe that the legal and cultural classification of psychotropic drugs as therapeutic medicines has made it difficult for us to understand how psychotropics are used to create new forms of social, psychic, and sexual death. While we are right to focus on the drug problems ravaging the American *human* population—problems with psychotropics, alcohol, opiates, cocaine, methamphetamines—we have to broaden our vision to include the drug problems experienced by American *institutions*. In fact, it is impossible for us to tackle our human drug problems without also confronting our institutional drug problems. To be clear, I am not saying that the suffering of real, flesh-and-blood human beings, so-called natural persons, is less important than our societal crisis. I am saying that these two problems are forever linked, and we will never solve one without solving the other. We have to be willing to view psychotropics through a necropolitical lens. Through psychotropics, the U.S. carceral state responds to and produces an affective or emotional situation in our society that works against psychic freedom. What affective or emotional social problems undergird the distribution of psychotropics in captive America? Using psychotropics to act on the psychic life spirit of people requires that state agents treat the spirit as if it is a material thing that can be forced into silence. Yet I still struggle to articulate *why* human beings, working as government agents and medical officers, forcibly drug other human beings into total psychic submission. Yes, committing spirit murder first requires having the right weapons. But what nerve, what unbridled feeling, what spiritual bankruptcy opens a person up to using these neurochemical weapons on imprisoned babies who have been separated from their parents? How do people come to care so little about the well-being of others that they become willing to kill their spirits by pressing psychotropics through their brains?

Fear, anger, and callous disregard are the cherished emotional children of settler colonialism, misogyny, and white supremacy. The affective world created by these feelings supersedes and supplants the rule of law, placing people of color, poor people, queer people, and the dispossessed squarely on the psychic chopping block. I can only speculate on what it must feel like to be in the body of one of the druggers, positioned to pacify the spirit of another human being. The internal monologue must go something like this: Because we fear and want to dispose of you, we are angry at you and at ourselves for feeling this way. Our disregard for you is because we fear you and cannot face ourselves for what we have done and continue to do to you. In the words of the great revolutionary Fannie Lou Hamer, "They know what they've done to us. All across this country. They know what they've done to us. This country is desperately sick."[13] So, disposable Others, your sadness and suffering is not worth our best biopharmaceutical investments. Perhaps the persistent belief in the innate dysfunctional brains floating within bodies marked by black and brown skin matters here. Even if we gave you these drugs, they wouldn't help you. You don't even have feelings that are worthy or recognizable with the gaze of our regard. *Animals don't feel, do they?* Do you even feel pain? In any case, you are already beyond retrieving. Do you even have a soul? Now, we have powerful tools with which to silence your cries, which we do not want to hear in the first place. We don't want to hear your babies cry. We don't want to hear you scream out on the streets when we accost you. Be silent and let us do what we will. Take your injections quietly.

ACKNOWLEDGMENTS

I feel an abiding sense of gratitude for the privilege of being able to write this book, a gift given to me by so many people and institutions. I would like to thank my wife, Rebekah, whose love for me, belief in me, and sacrifices for my vocation keep my fire burning bright. Our shared sense of mission to place our bodies, minds, and spirits in service of the least among us is a powerful source of energy and purpose for me. Our lifelong companionship has been and, God willing, will continue to be the bedrock of my life. I love you so very much. I also thank my two firecrackers, Ruth and Elias, for their love, humor, and uncanny ability to keep me grounded. I'm certain that my grandfathers, neither of whom is with me in the flesh but only in spirit, would probably laugh at the very possibility that their great-grandchildren would one day completely take for granted that their dad writes and publishes books. I am extremely fortunate to be in a position to give them that laugh.

I thank my wonderful parents, Charles and Christine Hatch, for their constant wraparound of support and unconditional love for my little family. I should have these people on a payroll somehow, given how good they are at promoting me and my ideas. I also give especially hearty thanks to Paula Bokros, my selfless other mother, who has fed, housed, and helped to take care of me for nearly thirty years. I offer my thanksgiving to my family circle (Sweet Nanny, Nicci, Stephani, Big Willie, Marcus, Aaron, Alison, Jackie, Christina, Cody, Briana, Cheyenne, Dakota, Alexis, and Elizabeth) for their love and encouragement. To my larger family circle, including James and all the good people in East Point and Hartford, my thanks for your love and faithfulness.

In my scholarly circle, I am grateful to many people who supported this project over the past ten years. First I thank Ronald Braithwaite and his fellows at the Morehouse School of Medicine for teaching me priceless lessons about research ethics and for providing the institutional context that gave rise to this project in its earliest formulations in the summer of 2009. I offer thanksgiving to Lesley Reid for pointing me to the truly excellent people in the Summer Research Institute of the Racial Democracy, Crime, and Justice Network (RDCJN): Ruth Peterson, Laurie Krivo, Dana Haynie, Townsand Price-Spratlen, Jason

Schnittker, Lori Burrington, Waverly Duck, Kishonna Gray, Mia Ortiz, LaDonna Long, Patrisia Macías-Rojas, Henrika McCoy, Delores Jones-Brown, Rod Brunson, Jody Miller, Robert Crutchfield, Stephanie DiPietro, Anthony Peguero, Evelyn Patterson, Reuben Miller, Eric Stewart, and Marjorie Zatz. Without their professional and scholarly guidance at a critical point in my life, this project would still be just a hunch.

I thank all my brilliant friends in and around the Science in Society Program at Wesleyan University for their intellectual collegiality: Joe Rouse, Jill Morawski, Jennifer Tucker, Paul Erickson, Bill Johnston, Lori Gruen, MJ Rubenstein, Mitali Thakor, Victoria Pitts-Taylor, Megan Glick, and Courtney Weiss Smith. Our program has been a generative force in the life of my mind and has given me an extraordinary opportunity to think through many of the issues I address in this book. Here, I have to thank two generations of Wesleyan students in my antipsychiatry lecture course and students in my Center for Prison Education seminar on the sociology of knowledge for walking through background material that informed my framing of this book. I offer special thanks to Marc Eisner, Liza McAlister, and the Center for African American Studies for their generous financial support for the publication of this book.

I thank all the folks who invited me to talk about this project with diverse audiences and whose questions, provocations, and behind-the-scenes support undoubtedly made it better: Jackie Orr, Lisa Jean Moore, Monica Casper, Laura Mamo, Emily Mann, Patrick Grzanka, Ruha Benjamin, Sydney Halpern, Kelly Moore, Joan Fujimora, Lundy Braun, and Ben Kail. Chris Vidmar, Haron Atkinson, and Victor Ogundipe provided valuable research assistance at Georgia State University. Substantial portions of this work were presented in the Department of Sociology at Syracuse University; in the Department of Criminal Justice at John Jay College; at the Black Studies and Biopolitics Seminar at Princeton University; at the conference "Speculative Visions of Race, Technology, Science, and Survival" at the University of California, Berkeley; in the Department of Sociology at the University of Maryland at College Park; at the "Inter/dependence" Medical Humanities Symposium at Rutgers University; at the Institute for Humanities Research at Arizona State University; and at the Wesleyan TEDx conference at Wesleyan University. Librarians at the Harry Ransom Center at the University of Texas at Austin helped me navigate the Jessica Mitford Papers. Librarians at the Bioethics Research Library at Georgetown

University helped me comb through the volumes of documents from the National Commission for the Protection of Human Subjects of Biomedical and Behavioral Research.

This work benefited from fruitful scholarly collaborations with Kym Bradley, Marik Xavier-Brier, Brandon Atell, and Eryn Viscarra. I am truly thankful for the boundless support of Jason Weidemann, whose editorial vision and ethical commitments to this work have brought it to life. Thank you to all the good people at the University of Minnesota Press whose labors put it on paper, especially my generous copy editor, Judy Selhorst, and to Lisa Guenther and an anonymous reviewer for their time, insights, and productive criticisms.

Finally, I offer a very special thanks to Renee M. Shelby, my co-author, friend, and comrade, for all of your work on *Silent Cells* over the years. This book would not have been possible without you. Any errors of fact or interpretation are my sole responsibility.

NOTES

PREFACE

1. In *Blood Sugar*, I critique the ways in which metabolic syndrome contributes to the naturalization of race and racial health inequality under conditions of color-blind scientific racism. Anthony Ryan Hatch, *Blood Sugar: Racial Pharmacology and Food Justice in Black America* (Minneapolis: University of Minnesota Press, 2016).

2. Michel Foucault, *Discipline and Punish: The Birth of the Prison* (London: Vintage Books, 1977).

3. "U.S. Sentencing Commission Unanimously Votes to Allow Delayed Retroactive Reduction in Drug Trafficking Sentences," U.S. Sentencing Commission, press release, July 18, 2014, https://www.ussc.gov.

INTRODUCTION

1. As of September 2015, according to the federal Adoption and Foster Care Analysis and Reporting System (AFCARS), there were 427,910 children in foster care across the United States. U.S. Department of Health and Human Services, Administration for Children and Families, Administration on Children, Youth and Families, Children's Bureau, *The AFCARS Report*, no. 23 (June 2016), https://www.acf.hhs.gov.

2. Erving Goffman, *Asylums: Essays on the Social Situation of Mental Patients and Other Inmates* (New York: Anchor Books, 1961); Tom Burns, *Erving Goffman* (London: Routledge, 1991).

3. Goffman, 6.

4. Goffman, 4–5.

5. Burns, *Erving Goffman*.

6. Goffman, *Asylums*, 12.

7. Goffman, 7.

8. Burns, *Erving Goffman*, 157.

9. Clifford L. Broman, "Race Differences in the Receipt of Mental Health Services among Young Adults," *Psychological Services* 9, no. 1 (2012): 38–48; Margarita Alegría, Pinka Chatterji, Kenneth Wells, Zhun Cao, Chih-nan Chen, David Takeuchi, James Jackson, and Xiao-Li Meng, "Disparity in Depression Treatment among Racial and Ethnic Minority Populations in the United States," *Psychiatric Services* 59, no. 11 (2008): 1264–72.

10. Ryne Paulose-Ram, Marc A. Safran, Bruce S. Jonas, Qiuping Gu, and Denise Orwig, "Trends in Psychotropic Medication Use among US Adults," *Pharmacoepidemiology and Drug Safety* 16, no. 5 (2007): 560–70; Qiuping Gu, Charles F. Dillon, and Vicki L. Burt, *Prescription Drug Use Continues to Increase: U.S. Prescription Drug Data for 2007–2008*, NCHS Data Brief, no. 42 (Hyattsville, Md.: National Center for Health Statistics, 2010); Laura A. Pratt, Debra J.

Brody, and Qiuping Gu, *Antidepressant Use in Persons Aged 12 and Over: United States, 2005–2008* (Hyattsville, Md.: National Center for Health Statistics, 2011); Bruce S. Jonas, Qiuping Gu, and Juan R. Albertorio-Diaz, *Psychotropic Medication Use among Adolescents: United States, 2005–2010,* NCHS Data Brief, no. 135 (Hyattsville, Md.: National Center for Health Statistics, 2013).

11. Thomas J. Moore and Donald R. Mattison, "Adult Utilization of Psychiatric Drugs and Differences by Sex, Age, and Race," *JAMA Internal Medicine* 177, no. 2 (2017): 274–75. The authors note that their estimate of long-term use is based on self-reported data limited to a single survey year.

12. Sherry A. Glied and Richard G. Frank, "Better but Not Best: Recent Trends in the Well-Being of the Mentally Ill," *Health Affairs* 28, no. 3 (2009): 637–48; Tami L. Mark, Katharine R. Levit, and Jeffrey A. Buck, "Datapoints: Psychotropic Drug Prescriptions by Medical Specialty," *Psychiatric Services* 60, no. 9 (2009): 1167; Ramin Mojtabai and Mark Olfson, "National Trends in Long-Term Use of Antidepressant Medications: Results from the US National Health and Nutrition Examination Survey," *Journal of Clinical Psychiatry* 75, no. 2 (2014): 169–77.

13. David Healy, Andrew Herxheimer, and David B. Menkes, "Antidepressants and Violence: Problems at the Interface of Medicine and Law," *PLOS Medicine* 3, no. 9 (2006): 1478–87; Thomas J. Moore, Joseph Glenmullen, and Curt D. Furberg, "Prescription Drugs Associated with Reports of Violence towards Others," *PLOS One* 5, no. 12 (2010): e15337; Peter R. Breggin, *Medication Madness: A Psychiatrist Exposes the Dangers of Mood-Altering Medications* (New York: St. Martin's Press, 2008); Peter R. Breggin, "Antidepressant-Induced Suicide, Violence, and Mania: Risks for Military Personnel," *Ethical Human Psychology and Psychiatry* 12, no. 2 (2010): 111–21.

14. Donald W. Light, "Bearing the Risks of Prescription Drugs," in *The Risks of Prescription Drugs,* ed. Donald W. Light (New York: Columbia University Press, 2010), 1–39; David Healy, *Pharmageddon* (Berkeley: University of California Press, 2012); Joseph Dumit, *Drugs for Life: How Pharmaceutical Companies Define Our Health* (Durham, N.C.: Duke University Press, 2012).

15. Hatch, *Blood Sugar*; Jonathan Kahn, *Race in a Bottle: The Story of BiDil and Racialized Medicine in a Post-genomic Age* (New York: Columbia University Press, 2013); Anne Pollock, *Medicating Race: Heart Disease and Durable Preoccupations with Difference* (Durham, N.C.: Duke University Press, 2012); Jackie Orr, *Panic Diaries: A Genealogy of Panic Disorder* (Durham, N.C.: Duke University Press, 2006); Jonathan Metzl, *Prozac on the Couch: Prescribing Gender in the Era of Wonder Drugs* (Durham, N.C.: Duke University Press, 2003).

16. Lauren E. Glaze, *Correctional Population in the United States, 2010,* BJS Bulletin, NCJ 236319 (Washington, D.C.: U.S. Department of Justice, Bureau of Justice Statistics, 2011).

17. E. Ann Carson, *Prisoners in 2016,* BJS Bulletin, NCJ 251149 (Washington, D.C.: U.S. Department of Justice, Bureau of Justice Statistics, 2018).

18. Ruth Wilson Gilmore, *Golden Gulag: Prisons, Surplus, Crisis, and Opposition in Globalizing California* (Berkeley: University of California Press, 2007).

19. Michelle Brown, *The Culture of Punishment: Prison, Society, and Spectacle*

(New York: New York University Press, 2009); Michael Welch, *Escape to Prison: Penal Tourism and the Pull of Punishment* (Berkeley: University of California Press, 2015); Dawn K. Cecil, *Prison Life in Popular Culture: From the Big House to "Orange Is the New Black"* (Boulder, Colo.: Lynne Rienner, 2015).

20. Douglass Shenson, Nancy Dubler, and David Michaels, "Jails and Prisons: The New Asylums?," *American Journal of Public Health* 80, no. 6 (1990): 655–56; E. Fuller Torrey, "Jails and Prisons: America's New Mental Hospitals," *American Journal of Public Health* 85, no. 12 (1995): 1611–13.

21. E. Fuller Torrey, Aaron D. Kennard, Don Eslinger, Richard Lamb, and James Pavle, *More Mentally Ill Persons Are in Jails and Prisons Than Hospitals: A Survey of the States* (Arlington, Va.: Treatment Advocacy Center, 2010).

22. Human Rights Watch, *Ill-Equipped: U.S. Prisons and Offenders with Mental Illness* (New York: Human Rights Watch, 2003).

23. Allen J. Beck and Laura M. Maruschak, *Mental Health Treatment in State Prisons, 2000*, BJS Special Report, NCJ 188215 (Washington, D.C.: U.S. Department of Justice, Bureau of Justice Statistics, 2001).

24. Andrew P. Wilper, Steffie Woolhandler, J. Wesley Boyd, Karen E. Lasser, Danny McCormick, David H. Bor, and David U. Himmelstein, "The Health and Health Care of U.S. Prisoners: Results of a Nationwide Survey," *American Journal of Public Health* 99, no. 4 (2009): 666–72.

25. "Vermont DOC: Nation's Biggest Dispenser of Psychotropic Medication," *Prison Legal News*, January 2008, https://www.prisonlegalnews.org/news.

26. Harley Lappin, testimony in *Human Rights at Home: Mental Illness in U.S. Prisons and Jails, Hearing before the Subcommittee on Human Rights and the Law, Committee on the Judiciary, U.S. Senate*, 111th Cong., 1st Sess. (September 15, 2009), https://www.gpo.gov/fdsys.

27. Torrey et al., *More Mentally Ill Persons Are in Jails*.

28. A. J. Gottschlich and G. Cetnar, "Drug Bills at Jail Top Food Costs," *Springfield (Ohio) News Sun*, August 20, 2002.

29. Tony Fabelo, *"Technocorrections": The Promises, the Uncertain Threats*, Research in Brief, NCJ 181411 (Washington, D.C.: U.S. Department of Justice, National Institute of Justice, 2000), https://www.ncjrs.gov.

30. Fabelo, 2, emphasis added.

31. Michael Massoglia, "Incarceration as Exposure: The Prison, Infectious Disease, and Other Stress-Related Illnesses," *Journal of Health and Social Behavior* 49, no. 1 (2008): 56–71.

32. Lorna Rhodes, *Total Confinement: Madness and Reason in the Maximum Security Prison* (Berkeley: University of California Press, 2004).

33. Jessica Mitford, *Kind and Usual Punishment: The Prison Business* (New York: Alfred A. Knopf, 1973).

34. For work in the 1970s, see Roy G. Spece, "Conditioning and Other Technologies Used to 'Treat?' 'Rehabilitate?' 'Demolish?' Prisoners and Mental Patients," *Southern California Law Review* 45, no. 2 (1972): 616–84; Michael H. Shapiro, "Legislating the Control of Behavior Control: Autonomy and the Coercive Use of Organic Therapies," *Southern California Law Review* 47, no. 2 (1974): 237–356; Richard Singer, "Consent of the Unfree: Medical Experimentation and

Behavior Modification in the Closed Institution, Part II," *Law and Human Behavior* 1, no. 2 (1977): 1–43. For somewhat more recent legal interpretations, see Jami Floyd, "The Administration of Psychotropic Drugs to Prisoners: State of the Law and Beyond," *California Law Review* 78 (1990): 1243–85; Kathleen Auerhahn and Elizabeth Dermody Leonard, "Docile Bodies? Chemical Restraints and the Female Inmate," *Journal of Criminal Law and Criminology* 90, no. 2 (2000): 599–634.

35. Douglas Del Paggio, "Psychotropic Medication Abuse by Inmates in Correctional Facilities," *Mental Health Clinician* 1, no. 8 (2012): 187–88; Joseph M. Pierre, Igor Shnayder, Donna A. Wirshing, and William C. Wirshing, "Intranasal Quetiapine Abuse," *American Journal of Psychiatry* 161, no. 9 (2004): 1718.

36. Ted Morgan, "Waiting for Justice—8th Floor: Homicides; 9th Floor: Addicts; 10th Floor: Suicidal: Entombed," *New York Times,* February 17, 1974.

37. Letter in Select Committee on Narcotics Abuse and Control, 96th Cong., 2nd Sess., *United States Bureau of Prisons Staff Study: Institutional Drug Abuse Treatment Programs and Utilization of Prescription Drugs at Five Institutions,* SCNAC-96-2-13 (Washington, D.C.: Government Printing Office, 1980), 89, emphasis added.

38. Lisa Guenther, *Solitary Confinement: Social Death and Its Afterlives* (Minneapolis: University of Minnesota Press, 2013); Rhodes, *Total Confinement.*

39. It has been well documented that black men have disproportionately fueled the expanding American prison population. In fact, as of December 13, 2013, nearly 3 percent of black men in the United States were incarcerated, compared to only 0.5 percent of white men. E. Ann Carson, *Prisoners in 2013,* BJS Bulletin, NCJ 247282 (Washington, D.C.: U.S. Department of Justice, Bureau of Justice Statistics, 2014). Given that African Americans make up only approximately 13 percent of the U.S. population, this disparity is breathtaking. However, what is often overlooked is that the fastest-rising demographic in prison is women. In 1980, there were 13,258 women in prison; by 2012, the number had risen to 113,605, almost a tenfold increase. As it is with men of color, women of color are disproportionately represented in American prisons. For details on these data, see E. Ann Carson and Daniela Golinelli, *Prisoners in 2012:* Trends in Admissions and Releases, 1991–2012, BJS Bulletin, NCJ 243920 (Washington, D.C.: U.S. Department of Justice, Bureau of Justice Statistics, 2013).

40. Patricia Williams, *The Alchemy of Race and Rights: Diary of a Law Professor* (Cambridge, Mass.: Harvard University Press, 1991); Patricia Hill Collins, *Black Sexual Politics: African Americans, Gender, and the New Racism* (New York: Routledge, 2005).

41. Intersectional frameworks, through which race, gender, sexuality, social class, disability, and nationality are viewed as intersecting axes of domination and resistance, shape these arguments by highlighting the ways in which systems of power draw on each other for meaning and operate simultaneously to maintain inequality and open up fissures for resistance. See Angela Y. Davis and Cassandra Shaylor, "Race, Gender, and the Prison Industrial Complex: California and Beyond," *Meridians: Feminism, Race, Transnationalism* 2, no. 1 (2001): 1–25; Julia Sudbury, ed., *Global Lockdown: Race, Gender, and the Prison–Industrial Complex*

(New York: Routledge, 2013); Jodie M. Lawston and Erica R. Meiners, "Ending Our Expertise: Feminists, Scholarship, and Prison Abolition," *Feminist Formations* 26, no. 2 (2014): 1–25.

42. Michelle Alexander, *The New Jim Crow: Mass Incarceration in the Age of Colorblindness* (New York: New Press, 2010); Angela Y. Davis, *Are Prisons Obsolete?* (New York: Seven Stories Press, 2003).

43. Elizabeth Ettore and Elianna Riska, *Gendered Moods: Psychotropics and Society* (London: Routledge, 1995).

44. Ira Sommers and Deborah R. Baskin, "The Prescription of Psychiatric Medications in Prison: Psychiatric versus Labeling Perspectives," *Justice Quarterly* 7, no. 4 (1990): 739–55; Clarice Feinman, *Women in the Criminal Justice System* (Westport, Conn.: Praeger, 1994); Barbara H. Zaitzow, "Psychotropic Control of Women Prisoners: The Perpetuation of Abuse of Imprisoned Women," *Justice Policy Journal* 7, no. 2 (2010): 1–37; Jennifer Kilty, "Governance through Psychiatrization: Seroquel and the New Prison Order," *Radical Psychology* 2, no. 7 (2008): 1–24.

45. Hilary Allen, "Rendering Them Harmless: The Professional Portrayal of Women Charged with Serious Violent Crimes," in *Criminology at the Crossroads: Feminist Readings in Crime and Justice,* ed. Kathleen Daly and Lisa Maher (New York: Oxford University Press, 1998), 54–68; Karlene Faith, *Unruly Women: The Politics of Confinement and Resistance* (New York: Seven Stories Press, 2011).

46. Charles H. Jones and Stephen M. Latimer, "*Liles v. Ward*: A Case Study in the Abuse of Psychotropic Drugs in Prison," *New England Journal of Prison Law* 8 (1982): 1–38.

47. Auerhahn and Leonard, "Docile Bodies?," 605.

48. Jones and Latimer, "*Liles v. Ward,*" 7.

49. Jacques Baillargeon and Salvador A. Contreras, "Antipsychotic Prescribing Patterns in the Texas Prison System," *Journal of the American Academy of Psychiatry and the Law* 29, no. 1 (2001): 48–53; Jacques Baillargeon, Sandra A. Black, Salvador A. Contreras, James Grady, and John Pulvino, "Anti-depressant Prescribing Patterns for Prison Inmates with Depressive Disorders," *Journal of Affective Disorders* 63, no. 1 (2001): 225–31.

50. Sullivan v. Flannigan and Parwatikar, 8 F.3d 591 (7th Cir. 1993).

51. Susan Leigh Star, "This Is Not a Boundary Object: Reflections on the Origin of a Concept," *Science, Technology, & Human Values* 35, no. 5 (2010): 601–17; Adriana Petryna, *Life Exposed: Biological Citizens after Chernobyl* (Princeton, N.J.: Princeton University Press, 2013).

52. Estelle v. Gamble, 429 U.S. 97 (1976); William J. Rold, "Thirty Years after Estelle v. Gamble: A Legal Retrospective," *Journal of Correctional Health Care* 14, no. 1 (2008): 11–20.

53. Centers for Medicare and Medicaid Services, *Code of Federal Regulations,* 483.13(a), https://www.gpo.gov/fdsys.

54. Texas Department of Family and Child Protective Services, "Rights of Children and Youth in Foster Care," Form K-908-2530, rev. March 2017, https://www.dfps.state.tx.us.

55. Floyd, "Administration of Psychotropic Drugs."

56. Lee Black, "Forced Medication of Prison Inmates," *Virtual Mentor* 10, no. 2 (2008): 106.

57. Washington v. Harper, 494 U. S. 219 (1990).

58. Sheldon Gelman, "The Biological Alteration Cases," *William and Mary Law Review* 36, no. 4 (1994): 1204.

59. Dennis Cichon, "The Right to Just Say No: A History and Analysis of the Right to Refuse Antipsychotic Drugs," *Los Angeles Law Review* 53 (1992): 283–426; Bruce J. Winick, "Psychotropic Medication and Competence to Stand Trial," *Law & Social Inquiry* 2, no. 3 (1977): 769–816; Patricia E. Sindel, "Fourteenth Amendment: The Right to Refuse Antipsychotic Drugs Masked by Prison Bars," *Journal of Criminal Law and Criminology* 81, no. 4 (1991): 952–80.

60. Riggins v. Nevada, 504 U.S. 127 (1992).

61. Sell v. United States, 539 U.S. 166 (2003).

62. Felce v. Fielder, 974 F.2d 1481 (1992).

63. Caitlin Steinke, "How the Medicate-to-Execute Scheme Undermines Individual Liberty, Offends Societal Norms, and Violates the Constitution," Hofstra Law Student Works, Paper 8 (2013); Howard V. Zonana, "Competency to Be Executed and Forced Medication: *Singleton v. Norris*," *Journal of the American Academy of Psychiatry and the Law* 31 (2003): 372–76.

64. Nelson v. Heyne, 491 F.2d 353 (7th Cir. 1974).

65. *Nelson*, 491 F.2d at 455.

66. *Nelson*, 491 F.2d at 456.

67. Edward M. Opton Jr., "Psychiatric Violence against Prisoners: When Therapy Is Punishment," *Mississippi Law Journal* 45, no. 3 (1974): 608.

68. Opton, 608.

69. Opton, 622.

70. See, for example, Auerhahn and Leonard, "Docile Bodies?"

71. Opton, "Psychiatric Violence against Prisoners," 639.

72. Opton, 640.

73. Opton, 640.

74. Singer, "Consent of the Unfree," 40.

75. First, I have collected federal, state, and local prison and jail performance audits of prison pharmacies and correctional health services. Second, I have collected publicly available government research reports and official policy statements that pertain to the mental health services currently provided in prison contexts. Third, I have collected original legal rulings and secondary scholarly interpretations of those rulings as they pertain to issues of state power, citizenship, and psychotropics in prison contexts. Finally, I have combed available journalistic accounts of the dynamics of psychotropic distribution in custodial institutions. Taken together, these primary materials enable me to provide historically nuanced interpretations of the meanings of psychotropics.

76. Patricia Williams, "Spirit-Murdering the Messenger: The Discourse of Fingerpointing as the Law's Response to Racism," *University of Miami Law Review* 42 (1987): 151.

77. Robin E. Sheriff, "Exposing Silence as Cultural Censorship: A Brazilian Case," *American Anthropologist* 102, no. 1 (2000): 114–32; Christina A. Sue, "He-

gemony and Silence: Confronting State-Sponsored Silences in the Field," *Journal of Contemporary Ethnography* 44, no. 1 (2015): 113–40; Robin Patric Clair, *Organizing Silence: A World of Possibilities* (Albany: State University of New York Press, 1998); Himika Bhattacharya, "Performing Silence: Gender, Violence, and Resistance in Women's Narratives from Lahaul, India," *Qualitative Inquiry* 15, no. 2 (2009): 359–71; Stefan Hirschauer, "Putting Things into Words: Ethnographic Description and the Silence of the Social," *Human Studies* 29, no. 4 (2007): 413–41.

78. Michel-Rolph Trouillot, *Silencing the Past: Power and the Production of History* (Boston: Beacon Press, 1995).

79. Paulo Freire, *Pedagogy of the Oppressed*, 50th anniversary ed. (New York: Bloomsbury Academic, 2018), 60.

80. James Scott, *Seeing Like a State: How Certain Schemes to Improve the Human Condition Have Failed* (New Haven, Conn.: Yale University Press, 1999); Aimé Césaire, *Discourse on Colonialism*, trans. Joan Pinkham (New York: Monthly Review Press, 2000).

81. Michel Foucault, *The History of Sexuality*, vol. 1, *An Introduction*, trans. R. Hurley (New York: Vintage Books, 1978); Michel Foucault, *"Society Must Be Defended": Lectures at the Collège de France, 1975–1976*, ed. Mauro Bertani and Alessandro Fontana, trans. David Macey (New York: Picador, 2003).

82. Achille Mbembe, "Necropolitics," *Public Culture* 15, no. 1 (2003): 14.

83. Giorgio Agamben, *State of Exception*, trans. Kevin Attell (Chicago: University of Chicago Press, 2005).

84. Mbembe, "Necropolitics," 40.

1. CLIMBING THE WALLS

1. Robert Proctor, *Agnotology: The Making and Unmaking of Ignorance* (Stanford, Calif.: Stanford University Press, 2008); Kristian H. Nielsen and Mads P. Sørensen, "How to Take Non-knowledge Seriously, or 'The Unexpected Virtue of Ignorance,'" *Public Understanding of Science* 26, no. 3 (2017): 385–92.

2. David E. Lilienfeld, "The First Pharmacoepidemiologic Investigations: National Drug Safety Policy in the United States, 1901–1902," *Perspectives in Biology and Medicine* 51, no. 2 (2008): 188–98; Brian L. Strom, Stephen E. Kimmel, and Sean Hennessy, eds., *Textbook of Pharmacoepidemiology* (Oxford: Wiley-Blackwell, 2013).

3. Adriana Petryna, *When Experiments Travel: Clinical Trials and the Global Search for Human Subjects* (Princeton, N.J.: Princeton University Press, 2009).

4. "Questions and Answers on FDA's Adverse Event Reporting System (FAERS)," U.S. Food and Drug Administration, updated June 4, 2018, https://www.fda.gov.

5. "FDA Adverse Event Reporting System (FAERS) Public Dashboard," U.S. Food and Drug Administration, updated July 23, 2018, https://www.fda.gov.

6. "Questions and Answers on FDA's Adverse Event Reporting System."

7. "Postmarket Drug and Biologic Safety Evaluations," U.S. Food and Drug Administration, updated October 6, 2017, https://www.fda.gov.

8. These include but are not limited to the National Household Survey

on Drug Abuse (1990–2001), the National Survey on Drug Use and Health (2002–current), the National Health and Nutrition Examination Survey (1959–current), and the Medical Expenditure Panel Survey (1996–current).

9. Geraldine Pierre, Roland J. Thorpe Jr., Gniesha Y. Dinwiddie, and Darrell J. Gaskin, "Are There Racial Disparities in Psychotropic Drug Use and Expenditures in a Nationally Representative Sample of Men in the United States? Evidence from the Medical Expenditure Panel Survey," *American Journal of Men's Health* 8, no. 1 (2014): 82–90; Broman, "Race Differences in the Receipt of Mental Health Services."

10. Paulose-Ram et al., "Trends in Psychotropic Medication Use."

11. Gail L. Daumit, Rosa M. Crum, Eliseo Guallar, Neil R. Powe, Annelle B. Primm, Donald M. Steinwachs, and Daniel E. Ford, "Outpatient Prescriptions for Atypical Antipsychotics for African Americans, Hispanics, and Whites in the United States," *Archives of General Psychiatry* 60, no. 2 (2003): 121–28.

12. Philip S. Wang, Joyce C. West, Terri Tanielian, and Harold Alan Pincus, "Recent Patterns and Predictors of Antipsychotic Medication Regimens Used to Treat Schizophrenia and Other Psychotic Disorders," *Schizophrenia Bulletin* 26, no. 2 (2000): 451–57.

13. Tracy L. Skaer, David A. Sclar, Linda M. Robison, and Richard S. Galin, "Trends in the Rate of Depressive Illness and Use of Antidepressant Pharmacotherapy by Ethnicity/Race: An Assessment of Office-Based Visits in the United States, 1992–1997," *Clinical Therapeutics* 22, no. 12 (2000): 1575–89; Alexander S. Young, Ruth Klap, Cathy D. Sherbourne, and Kenneth B. Wells, "The Quality of Care for Depressive and Anxiety Disorders in the United States," *Archives of General Psychiatry* 58, no. 1 (2001): 55–61; Amy M. Kilbourne and Harold Alan Pincus, "Patterns of Psychotropic Medication Use by Race among Veterans with Bipolar Disorder," *Psychiatric Services* 57, no. 1 (2006): 123–26.

14. Baillargeon and Contreras, "Antipsychotic Prescribing Patterns"; Baillargeon et al., "Anti-depressant Prescribing Patterns."

15. Baillargeon et al., "Anti-depressant Prescribing Patterns."

16. Elise V. Griffiths, Jon Willis, and M. Joy Spark, "A Systematic Review of Psychotropic Drug Prescribing for Prisoners," *Australian and New Zealand Journal of Psychiatry* 46, no. 5 (2012): 407–21.

17. Emil R. Pinta and Robert E. Taylor, "Quetiapine Addiction?," *American Journal of Psychiatry* 164, no. 1 (2007): 174; Rusty Reeves, Herbert H. Kaldany, Jordan Lieberman, and Rajiv Vyas, "Creation of a Metabolic Monitoring Program for Second-Generation (Atypical) Antipsychotics," *Journal of Correctional Health Care* 15 (2009): 292–301. In my own work, I have analyzed the ways in which metabolic syndrome has been used to capture the negative side effects of second-generation, atypical antipsychotics—high blood sugar, high cholesterol, and excessive weight gain. See Hatch, *Blood Sugar.*

18. Stephanie Minor-Harper, *State and Federal Prisoners, 1925–85,* BJS Bulletin, NCJ 102494 (Washington, D.C.: U.S. Department of Justice, Bureau of Justice Statistics, 1986), https://www.ncjrs.gov.

19. In 1979, 11,397 inmates were successfully interviewed in 215 prisons; in

1986, 13,711 inmates were interviewed in 275 prisons; and in 1991, 13,986 inmates were interviewed in 272 prisons.

20. Paula M. Ditton, *Mental Health and Treatment of Inmates and Probationers*, BJS Special Report, NCJ 174463 (Washington, D.C.: U.S. Department of Justice, Bureau of Justice Statistics, 1999), 2, http://www.bjs.gov.

21. Doris J. James and Lauren E. Glaze, *Mental Health Problems of Prison and Jail Inmates*, BJS Special Report, NCJ 213600 (Washington, D.C.: U.S. Department of Justice, Bureau of Justice Statistics, 2006), http://www.bjs.gov.

22. Detailed symptom data suggest that between 2.3 percent and 3.9 percent of the prisoners surveyed were diagnosed with schizophrenia or other psychotic disorders, with symptoms including hallucinations, delusions, and disorganized speech and behavior. Between 13.1 percent and 18.6 percent suffered from major depression, with symptoms including appetite or weight change, changes in sleep, decreased energy, feelings of worthlessness or guilt, and difficulty thinking, concentrating, or making decisions; of this group, 15 percent ultimately committed suicide. Between 2.1 percent and 4.3 percent were diagnosed with bipolar disorder, with symptoms including rapidly alternating moods such as sadness, irritability, and euphoria. Suicide rates for those with this disorder ranged between 10 percent and 15 percent. Between 22 percent and 30 percent of the prisoners surveyed were diagnosed with anxiety disorders, such as panic disorder, agoraphobia, obsessive-compulsive disorder, posttraumatic stress disorder, and general anxiety disorder.

23. James and Glaze, *Mental Health Problems*, 3.

24. Wilper et al., "The Health and Health Care of U.S. Prisoners."

25. Ditton, *Mental Health and Treatment*.

26. Jennifer Bronson and Marcus Berzofsky, *Indicators of Mental Health Problems Reported by Prisoners and Jail Inmates, 2011–12*, BJS Special Report, NCJ 250612 (Washington, D.C.: U.S. Department of Justice, Bureau of Justice Statistics, 2017).

27. Beck and Maruschak, *Mental Health Treatment in State Prisons*, 1. The census included prisons and penitentiaries; boot camps; prison farms; reception, diagnostic, and classification centers; road campuses; forestry and conservation camps; youthful offender facilities (except in California); vocational training facilities; prison hospitals; drug and alcohol treatment facilities; and state-operated local detention facilities (in Alaska, Connecticut, Delaware, Hawaii, Rhode Island, and Vermont).

28. "National Survey of Prison Health Care," National Center for Health Statistics, Centers for Disease Control and Prevention, updated August 26, 2016, https://www.cdc.gov.

29. Marguerite J. Ro, Carolina Casares, Henrie M. Treadwell, and Kisha Braithwaite, "Access to Mental Health Care and Substance Abuse Treatment for Men of Color in the U.S.: Findings from the National Healthcare Disparities Report," *Challenge* 12, no. 2 (2006): 65–74.

30. See, for example, Zaitzow, "Psychotropic Control of Women Prisoners."

2. THE PHARMACY PRISON

1. Charles L. Pickens, "Pharmacy in Prison," *Journal of Pharmaceutical Sciences* 26, no. 1 (1936): 54.

2. Pickens, 55.

3. Pickens, 55, emphasis added.

4. Pickens, 57. On prisons as tourist destinations, see Welch, *Escape to Prison*; on prisons as sites of cultural production more broadly, see Brown, *The Culture of Punishment*.

5. "About Us," Minnesota Multistate Coordinating Alliance for Pharmacy, http://www.mmd.admin.state.mn.us.

6. Office of the Legislative Auditor, State of Minnesota, *Health Services in State Correctional Facilities* (St. Paul: State of Minnesota, 2014), 89.

7. Minnesota Multistate Coordinating Alliance for Pharmacy, "Prescription Filling and Pharmacy Services Addendum #2," June 9, 2017, http://www.bidnet.com/bneattachments?/453772112.pdf.

8. "About Us," Minnesota Multistate Coordinating Alliance for Pharmacy.

9. "About Corizon Health: Partner Locations," Corizon Health, http://www.corizonhealth.com.

10. "PharmaCorr: Information on Services," Corizon Health, http://www.corizonpharmacy.com.

11. Greg Dober, "Corizon Needs a Checkup: Problems with Privatized Correctional Healthcare," *Prison Legal News,* March 2014, https://www.prisonlegalnews.org.

12. Anthony Ryan Hatch, "Billions Served: Prison Food Regimes, Nutritional Punishment, and Gastronomical Resistance," in *Captivating Technology: Race, Carceral Technoscience, and Liberatory Imagination in Everyday Life,* ed. Ruha Benjamin (Durham, N.C.: Duke University Press, 2019).

13. Pew Charitable Trusts and John D. and Catherine T. MacArthur Foundation, *State Prison Health Care Spending: An Examination* (Philadelphia: Pew Charitable Trusts and MacArthur Foundation, 2014), http://www.pewtrusts.org.

14. The ten states were Florida, Illinois, Minnesota, Nebraska, Ohio, Oregon, Pennsylvania, Rhode Island, Utah, and Washington.

15. Chad Kinsella, *Corrections Health Care Costs* (Lexington, Ky.: Council of State Governments, 2004), 3.

16. Kinsella, 16.

17. *Department of Corrections Healthcare: Public Health and Public Safety in the Commonwealth's Prisons* (Harrisburg, Pa.: Coalition for Labor Engagement and Accountable Revenues and SEIUHealthcare, 2011), 3.

18. James Austin and Garry Coventry, *Emerging Issues on Privatized Prisons,* NCCD Monograph, NCJ 181249 (Washington, D.C.: U.S. Department of Justice, Bureau of Justice Assistance, 2001), https://www.ncjrs.gov.

19. "ICON Minimum Data Entry Requirements for Institutions," Iowa Department of Corrections, last revised December 2016, https://doc.iowa.gov.

20. "District Policies," Fifth Judicial District, Iowa Department of Correctional Services, http://fifthdcs.com.

21. *FY2012 Annual Report,* Iowa Department of Corrections, 2012, 88.

22. *Department of Corrections, Internal Health Care Provided to Inmates,* performance audit, Office of the State Auditor, Colorado, September 2005, 48 (hereafter cited as Colorado audit).

23. Colorado audit, 52.

24. Colorado audit, 53.

25. *Division of Prisons—Central Pharmacy Inventory,* performance audit, Office of the State Auditor, North Carolina, December 2009, 1.

26. *Performance Audit: Jail Health Services' Pharmacy Operations and Medication Management,* King County Auditor's Office, Report No. 2007-04, October 2007, iii (hereafter cited as King County audit).

27. King County audit, 15.

28. *Correctional Health Care: Annual Cost Overruns, but Contract Oversight Has Improved,* Office of the State Auditor, Vermont, October 24, 2013, 17 (hereafter cited as Vermont audit).

29. Vermont audit, 19.

30. Vermont audit, 21.

31. *Mental Health in New Hampshire Correctional Facilities: Costs and Quality of Care,* PRS Policy Brief 0708-11, Policy Research Shop, Rockefeller Center at Dartmouth College, June 30, 2008 (hereafter cited as New Hampshire audit).

32. New Hampshire audit, 2.

33. New Hampshire audit, 3.

34. New Hampshire audit, 1.

35. New Hampshire audit, 9.

36. *A Performance Audit of the Salt Lake County Adult Detention Center Pharmaceutical Operation,* Salt Lake County Auditor's Office, May 2007, 8 (hereafter cited as Salt Lake County audit).

37. Salt Lake County audit, 8. I cannot verify the name of this contractor, but I believe it to be MHM Services, Inc., headquartered in Vienna, Virginia. This company took over jail operations in Salt Lake County in November 2003. MHM Services claims that it is "the leading national provider of mental health services for correctional systems." "About," MHM Services, Inc., http://www.mhm-services.com.

38. Salt Lake County audit, 10.

39. Salt Lake County audit, 48.

40. *Allegany County: County Jail Payroll and Inmate Prescription Medications,* Division of Local Government and School Accountability, Office of the New York State Comptroller, January 2014, 18 (hereafter cited as Allegany County audit).

41. Allegany County audit, 25.

42. *An Evaluation of Prison Health Care, Department of Corrections,* Legislative Audit Bureau, Wisconsin, May 2001, 3 (hereafter cited as Wisconsin audit, 2001).

43. "Taycheedah Inmate Dies after Pleading for Help," *Journal Times* (Racine, Wis.), February 16, 2000, http://journaltimes.com.

44. Wisconsin audit, 2001, 22. The eleven drugs (and their total costs and ranks in the list) were Seroquel ($593,164, number 1), Risperdal ($553,531, number 2), Paxil ($349,752, number 3), Zoloft ($242,289, number 4), Neurontin

($225,735, number 6), Depakote ($219,542, number 8), Prozac ($215,571, number 9), Zyprexa ($204,398, number 10), Buspar ($109,342, number 17), Remeron ($104,051, number 18), and Celexa ($83,285, number 20).

45. Wisconsin audit, 2001, 53.

46. *An Evaluation: Inmate Mental Health Care, Department of Corrections, Department of Health Services,* Legislative Audit Bureau, Wisconsin, Report 09-4, March 2009, 19 (hereafter cited as Wisconsin audit, 2009).

47. Wisconsin audit, 2009, 19.

48. Wisconsin audit, 2009, 11.

49. Wisconsin audit, 2009, 12.

50. Wisconsin audit, 2009, 45.

51. Wisconsin audit, 2009, 19–20.

52. Wisconsin audit, 2009, 27.

53. Wisconsin audit, 2009, 42.

54. Wisconsin audit, 2009, 27.

55. Wisconsin audit, 2001, 46.

56. *Performance Audit of Pharmaceutical Costs, Department of Corrections,* Office of the Auditor General, Michigan, March 2011, 43 (hereafter cited as Michigan audit).

57. Michigan audit, 13.

58. Michigan audit, 62.

59. Michigan audit, 15.

60. Michigan audit, 45.

61. Michigan audit, 16.

62. *Special Report: Lost Opportunities for Savings within California Prison Pharmacies,* Office of the Inspector General, California, April 2010, 1 (hereafter cited as California audit).

63. California audit, 1.

64. California audit, 5.

65. California audit, 6–7.

66. California audit, 2.

67. California audit, 1.

68. California audit, 14.

69. California audit, 20.

70. California audit, 20.

71. California audit, 20.

72. California audit, 25.

73. *Audit of the Federal Bureau of Prisons Pharmacy Services,* U.S. Department of Justice, Office of the Inspector General, Audit Division, November 2005, 1 (hereafter cited as BOP audit, 2005).

74. This audit was carried out at the BOP headquarters and at twelve BOP institutions: Alderson Federal Prison Camp in West Virginia, Atlanta U.S. Penitentiary (USP) in Georgia, Atwater USP in California, Danbury Federal Correctional Institution (FCI) in Connecticut, Florence Administrative Maximum Facility in Colorado, Florence FCI in Colorado, Florence USP in Colorado, Forrest City FCI in New Mexico, La Tuna FCI in New Mexico, Oklahoma City Federal

Transfer Center in Oklahoma, Oxford FCI in Wisconsin, and Springfield Medical Center in Missouri.

75. BOP audit, 2005, iv.

76. BOP audit, 2005, 8.

77. BOP audit, 2005, 7.

78. BOP audit, 2005, 7.

79. "We found that the BOP pharmacies were not always in compliance with applicable BOP policies and procedures. . . . We found that 384 (35 percent) of the prescriptions reviewed were not in compliance with BOP policy. Specifically we found prescriptions for which: (1) the pharmacist's or physician's signature was not documented; (2) the separate written prescription form for controlled substances was not maintained; (3) required information was missing in inmates' medical files; (4) controlled substance prescription forms were missing a DEA registration number or required signature; and (5) the prescription time period exceeded the BOP policy for controlled substances." BOP audit, 2005, 50.

80. BOP audit, 2005, 48.

81. *Health Services in State Correctional Facilities,* Program Evaluation Division, Office of the Legislative Auditor, Minnesota, February 2014, 88 (hereafter cited as Minnesota audit).

82. Minnesota audit, 88.

83. Minnesota audit, 88–89.

84. Minnesota audit, 89.

3. EXPERIMENTAL PATRIOTS

1. Specifically, I interrogate (1) *Prisons, Inmates, and Drug Testing,* the summary report of the Conference on Drug Research in Prisons, August 6–8, 1973, sponsored by the Pharmaceutical Manufacturers Association (PMA) and the National Council on Crime and Delinquency (NCCD); (2) the PMA's "Statement of Principles on the Conduct of Pharmaceutical Research in the Prison Environment, February 11, 1975"; and (3) Parke, Davis and Company's 1975 "Policy on the Use of Humans as Subjects in Clinical Investigation in an Institutional Setting." All of these documents are found in the Archival Collection of the National Commission for the Protection of Human Subjects of Biomedical and Behavioral Research, 1974–1978, Georgetown Bioethics Research Library, Washington, D.C.

2. See Jon M. Harkness, "Research behind Bars: A History of Nontherapeutic Experimentation on American Prisoners" (PhD diss., University of Wisconsin–Madison, 1996); Jon Harkness, "Nuremberg and the Issue of Wartime Experiments on U.S. Prisoners," *Journal of the American Medical Association* 276, no. 20 (1996): 1672–75; Allen Hornblum and Osagie K. Obasogie, "Medical Exploitation: Inmates Must Not Become Guinea Pigs Again," *Philadelphia Inquirer,* September 13, 2007; Jonathan Moreno, *Undue Risk: Secret State Experiments on Humans* (New York: W. H. Freeman, 2000).

3. National Commission for the Protection of Human Subjects of Biomedical and Behavioral Research, "Research Involving Prisoners," staff paper (Washington, D.C., 1975), 2, Archival Collection of the National Commission

for the Protection of Human Subjects of Biomedical and Behavioral Research, 1974–1978, Georgetown Bioethics Research Library, Washington, D.C.

4. Michael Mills and Norval Morris, "Prisoners as Laboratory Animals," *Society* 11, no. 5 (1974): 60; Mitford, *Kind and Usual Punishment*.

5. National Commission for the Protection of Human Subjects, "Research Involving Prisoners," 31.

6. Robert Mitchell and Catherine Waldby, "National Biobanks: Clinical Labor, Risk Production, and the Creation of Biovalue," *Science, Technology, & Human Values* 35, no. 3 (2010): 330–55.

7. James H. Jones, *Bad Blood: The Tuskegee Syphilis Experiment* (New York: Free Press, 1993); Harriet A. Washington, *Medical Apartheid: The Dark History of Medical Experimentation on Black Americans from Colonial Times to the Present* (New York: Doubleday, 2006).

8. Washington, *Medical Apartheid*.

9. Allen M. Hornblum, *Acres of Skin: Human Experiments at Holmesburg Prison* (New York: Routledge, 1998).

10. *Trials of War Criminals before the Nuernberg Military Tribunals under Control Council Law No. 10*, vol. 2, *The Medical Case* (Washington, D.C.: Government Printing Office, 1949).

11. National Commission for the Protection of Human Subjects, "Research Involving Prisoners," 3.

12. American Medical Association, "Supplementary Report of the Judicial Council, Proceedings of the House of Delegates Annual Meeting, 9–11 December," *Journal of the American Medical Association* 132, no. 1090 (1946).

13. Quoted in Douglas O. Linder, "The Nuremberg Trials: The Doctors Trial," Famous Trials, http://www.famous-trials.com.

14. *Trials of War Criminals before the Nuernberg Military Tribunals*, 181. Article 1 of the Nuremberg Code states: "The voluntary consent of the human subject is absolutely essential. This means that the person involved should have legal capacity to give consent; should be so situated as to be able to exercise free power of choice, without the intervention of any element of force, fraud, deceit, duress, over-reaching, or other ulterior form of constraint or coercion; and should have sufficient knowledge and comprehension of the elements of the subject matter involved as to enable him to make an understanding and enlightened decision."

15. George J. Annas and Michael A. Grodin, *The Nazi Doctors and the Nuremberg Code: Human Rights in Human Experimentation* (New York: Oxford University Press, 1992).

16. Rebecca Lowen, "Memorandum to ACHRE from Rebecca Lowen, Consultant to the Advisory Committee: Discussion of the Ethics of Human Experimentation in the Medical and Scientific Literature," Advisory Committee on Human Radiation Experiments (Washington, D.C., 1995), 1, http://www2.gwu.edu/~nsarchiv.

17. Harkness, "Nuremberg and the Issue of Wartime Experiments."

18. Quoted in Maurice H. Pappworth, *Human Guinea Pigs: Experimentation on Man* (New York: Routledge & Kegan Paul, 1967), 64.

19. Irving Ladimer, "Human Experimentation: Mediolegal Aspects," *New England Journal of Medicine* 257 (1957): 18–24; Henry K. Beecher, "Ethics and Clinical Research," *New England Journal of Medicine* 24, no. 274 (1966): 1354–60; Pappworth, *Human Guinea Pigs*; Mitford, *Kind and Usual Punishment*.

20. Ladimer, "Human Experimentation"; Beecher, "Ethics and Clinical Research"; Maurice H. Pappworth, "Human Guinea Pigs: A History," *British Medical Journal* 301, no. 6766 (1990): 1456.

21. These exposés included revelations about the Sloan-Kettering Cancer Studies at the Jewish Chronic Disease Hospital in 1964, the Tuskegee Syphilis Study in 1972, experimental brain psychosurgery at the Vacaville Prison in California in 1972, and dozens of other unethical studies. See Beecher, "Ethics and Clinical Research"; Pappworth, *Human Guinea Pigs*; Mitford, *Kind and Usual Punishment*.

22. National Commission for the Protection of Human Subjects of Biomedical and Behavioral Research, *The Belmont Report: Ethical Principles and Guidelines for the Protection of Human Subjects of Research* (Washington, D.C.: U.S. Department of Health, Education, and Welfare, 1979).

23. *Prisons, Inmates, and Drug Testing*, 5.

24. *Prisons, Inmates, and Drug Testing*, 8.

25. *Prisons, Inmates, and Drug Testing*, 5.

26. *Prisons, Inmates, and Drug Testing*, 9, emphasis added.

27. *Prisons, Inmates, and Drug Testing*, 16.

28. *Prisons, Inmates, and Drug Testing*, 6.

29. *Prisons, Inmates, and Drug Testing*, 21.

30. *Prisons, Inmates, and Drug Testing*, 18.

31. *Prisons, Inmates, and Drug Testing*, 14.

32. *Prisons, Inmates, and Drug Testing*, 18, 21, 23.

33. Parke-Davis, "Policy on the Use of Humans as Subjects," 1.

34. PMA, "Statement of Principles on the Conduct of Pharmaceutical Research," 1–2.

35. PMA, 2.

36. National Commission for the Protection of Human Subjects, "Research Involving Prisoners," 29.

37. See, for example, Moreno, *Undue Risk*.

38. National Minority Conference on Human Experimentation, "Summary of Plenary Sessions and Workshop Sessions: The Use of Prisoners in Human Experimentation," National Commission Papers (Washington, D.C., 1976), 3.

39. National Commission for the Protection of Human Subjects of Biomedical and Behavioral Research, *Research Involving Prisoners: Report and Recommendations*, DHEW Publication No. (OS) 76-131 (Washington, D.C.: Government Printing Office, 1976), 36.

40. Harkness, "Research behind Bars," 2.

41. Harkness, 208.

42. Stephen Gettinger and Kevin Krajick, "The Demise of Prison Medical Research," *Corrections Magazine* 5, no. 4 (1979): 4–14; Kevin Krajick and F. Moriarty, "Life in the Lab: Safer Than the Cellblocks?," *Corrections Magazine* 5, no. 4

(1979): 15–20; Marjorie Sun, "Inmates Sue to Keep Research in Prisons," *Science* 212, no. 4495 (May 8, 1981), 650–51.

43. National Commission for the Protection of Human Subjects, "Research Involving Prisoners."

44. Irvin Gilchrist, ed., *Medical Experimentation on Prisoners Must Stop! Documents Generated during the Course of a Struggle* (College Park, Md.: Urban Information Interpreters, 1974), 7.

45. Leslie Berger and Mary Lee Bundy, *Secrecy and Medical Experimentation on Prisoners: A Case Study of the Role of Government Information Suppression in the Repression and Exploitation of People* (College Park, Md.: Urban Information Interpreters, 1974), 32.

46. Berger and Bundy, 15.

47. T. C. Smith to G. D. Wood, "Volunteer Research Populations, State Prison of Southern Michigan," Parke-Davis interoffice memorandum, January 8, 1975, Archival Collection of the National Commission for the Protection of Human Subjects of Biomedical and Behavioral Research, 1974–1978, Georgetown Bioethics Research Library, Washington, D.C.

48. Lawrence O. Gostin, Cori Vanchieri, and Andrew Pope, eds., *Ethical Considerations for Research Involving Prisoners* (Washington, D.C.: National Academies Press, 2006), ix–x.

49. Gostin et al., xii.

50. Gostin et al., xii.

51. Gregory Dober, "Cheaper Than Chimpanzees: Expanding the Use of Prisoners in Medical Experiments," *Prison Legal News*, March 2008, 1–17; Barron Lerner, "Subjects or Objects? Prisoners and Human Experimentation," *New England Journal of Medicine* 356, no. 18 (2007): 1806; Keramet Reiter, "Experimentation on Prisoners: Persistent Dilemmas in Rights and Regulations," *California Law Review* 97, no. 2 (2009): 501–66.

52. "Declaration of Helsinki 2008," World Medical Association, October 2008, https://www.wma.net.

53. Institute of Medicine, Report Brief for *Ethical Considerations for Research Involving Prisoners*, June 2006.

54. Berger and Bundy, *Secrecy and Medical Experimentation*, 34.

4. PSYCHIC STATES OF EMERGENCY

1. Dana Ziegler, "Race, Mental Illness, and Kamilah Brock," *Michigan Journal of Race & Law* 21 (September 29, 2015), https://mjrl.org.

2. Kamilah Brock v. The City of New York, New York City Health and Hospitals Corporation, Harlem Hospital, Dr. Elizabeth Lescouflair, Dr. Zana Doubroshi, Dr. Alan Dudley Labor, and New York City Police Officers John Doe 1–3, U.S. District Court, Southern District of New York, Complaint Case 1:15-cv-01832-VSB, filed March 12, 2015.

3. Alisa Lincoln, "Psychiatric Emergency Room Decision-Making, Social Control and the 'Undeserving Sick,'" *Sociology of Health & Illness* 28, no. 1 (2006): 54–75.

4. Agamben, *State of Exception*.

5. Ornulv Odegard, "Pattern of Discharge from Norwegian Psychiatric Hospitals before and after the Introduction of the Psychotropic Drugs," *American Journal of Psychiatry* 120, no. 8 (1964): 772–78; Andrew Scull, *Decarceration: Community Treatment and the Deviant—A Radical View* (Englewood Cliffs, N.J.: Prentice Hall, 1977).

6. William Gronfein, "Psychotropic Drugs and the Origins of Deinstitutionalization," *Social Problems* 32, no. 5 (1985): 437–54.

7. E. Fuller Torrey, *American Psychosis: How the Federal Government Destroyed the Mental Illness Treatment System* (New York: Oxford University Press, 2014), 33.

8. Richard G. Frank, Rena M. Conti, and Howard H. Goldman, "Mental Health Policy and Psychotropic Drugs," *Milbank Quarterly* 83, no. 2 (2005): 271–98.

9. George Paulson, *Closing the Asylums: Causes and Consequences of the Deinstitutionalization Movement* (Jefferson, N.C.: McFarland, 2012); Lisa Davis, Anthony Fulginiti, Liat Kriegel, and John S. Brekke, "Deinstitutionalization? Where Have All the People Gone?," *Current Psychiatry Reports* 14, no. 3 (2012): 259–69.

10. Glied and Frank, "Better but Not Best."

11. Carol A. B. Warren, "New Forms of Social Control: The Myth of Deinstitutionalization," *American Behavioral Scientist* 24, no. 6 (1981): 726. See also Phil Brown, *The Transfer of Care: Psychiatric Deinstitutionalization and Its Aftermath* (New York: Routledge, 1985); Leona Bachrach, *Deinstitutionalization: An Analytical Review and Sociological Perspective* (Washington, D.C.: National Institute of Mental Health, 1976).

12. Joseph P. Morrissey and Howard H. Goldman, "Care and Treatment of the Mentally Ill in the United States: Historical Developments and Reforms," *Annals of the American Academy of Political and Social Science* 484 (March 1986): 12–27.

13. *Deinstitutionalization of the Mentally Ill, Hearings before the Subcommittee on Fiscal Affairs and Health of the Committee on the District of Columbia, U.S. House of Representatives*, 97th Cong. (November 2, 17–18, 1981); *Deinstitutionalization, Mental Illness, and Medications, Hearing before the Committee on Finance, U.S. Senate*, 103rd Cong., 2nd Sess. (May 10, 1994).

14. John Snowdon, Susan Day, and Wesley Baker, "Current Use of Psychotropic Medication in Nursing Homes," *International Psychogeriatrics* 18, no. 2 (2006): 241–50.

15. Misty Stenslie, testimony in *Prescription Psychotropic Drug Use among Children in Foster Care, Hearing before the Subcommittee on Income Security and Family Support of the Committee on Ways and Means, U.S. House of Representatives*, 110th Cong., 2nd Sess. (May 8, 2008), 51.

16. *Exploring the Relationship between Medication and Veteran Suicide, Hearing before the Committee on Veterans Affairs, U.S. House of Representatives*, 111th Cong., 2nd Sess. (February 24, 2010).

17. Lukasz Kamienski, *Shooting Up: A Short History of Drugs and War* (New York: Oxford University Press, 2016).

18. Peter R. Breggin, "Military to Hold Conference on Escalating Suicides; Drugs Not Allowed," Huffington Post, June 21, 2012, http://www.huffingtonpost .com/dr-peter-breggin/military-suicide_b_1602927.html.

19. Brett Schneider, John C. Bradley, and David M. Benedek, "Psychiatric Medications for Deployment: An Update," Military Medicine 172, no. 7 (2007): 685. See also Kenneth D. Marshall and Kathryn L. Hall-Boyer, "Military Objectives versus Patient Interests," in Ethical Problems in Emergency Medicine: A Discussion-Based Review, ed. John Jesus and Peter Rosen (Chichester: John Wiley, 2012), 247–58.

20. Schneider et al., "Psychiatric Medications for Deployment," 681–85; Robert M. Bray, Michael R. Pemberton, Marian E. Lane, Laurel L. Hourani, Mark J. Mattiko, and Lorraine A. Babeu, "Substance Use and Mental Health Trends among US Military Active Duty Personnel: Key Findings from the 2008 DoD Health Behavior Survey," Military Medicine 175, no. 6 (2010): 390–99.

21. Bob Brewin, "Military's Drug Policy Threatens Troops' Health, Doctors Say," NextGov, January 18, 2011, https://www.nextgov.com. See also Bridget M. Kuehn, "Military Probes Epidemic of Suicide," Journal of the American Medical Association 304, no. 13 (2010): 1427–30.

22. James Dao, Benedict Carey, and Dan Frosch, "For Some Troops, Powerful Drug Cocktails Have Deadly Results," New York Times, February 13, 2011.

23. Jeremey Schwartz, "Soaring Cost of Military Drugs Could Hurt Budget," Austin American-Statesman, December 29, 2012, https://www.statesman.com.

24. Andrew Tilghman and Brendan McGarry, "Medicating the Military: Use of Psychiatric Drugs Has Spiked; Concerns Surface About Suicide, Other Dangers," Army Times, March 17, 2010.

25. Michael Norman Knowlan, Juan Carlos Arguello, and Frances Irene Stewart, "A Survey of Navy Physicians' Attitudes toward the Use of Selective Serotonin Reuptake Inhibitors in Active Duty Military Personnel," Military Medicine 166, no. 6 (2001): 526–29.

26. William H. Grant and Phillip J. Resnick, "Right of Active Duty Military Personnel to Refuse Psychiatric Treatment," Behavioral Sciences and the Law 7, no. 3 (1989): 339–54.

27. Kim Murphy, "Soldiers at War in Fog of Psychotropic Drugs," Seattle Times, April 9, 2012, http://seattletimes.com; Amy Willis, "Prescribed Drugs 'to Blame over Spate of Violence among US Soldiers,'" Telegraph, April 9, 2012, http://www.telegraph.co.uk.

28. Robert Burns, "Military Suicides Reach a Record High," Durango Herald, January 13, 2013.

29. U.S. Department of Veterans Affairs, Office of Suicide Prevention, Suicide among Veterans and Other Americans (Washington, D.C.: U.S. Department of Veterans Affairs, 2016).

30. Dao et al., "For Some Troops."

31. Heather Clark, "Fort Campbell's Warrior Care Clinic Offers Integrative Therapies," Fort Campbell Courier, January 27, 2012, http://www.army.mil.

32. Timothy B. Jeffrey, Robert J. Rankin, and Louise K. Jeffrey, "In Service of Two Masters: The Ethical-Legal Dilemma Faced by Military Psychologists,"

Professional Psychology: Research and Practice 23, no. 2 (1992): 91; Ilan Zrihen, Isaac Ashkenazi, Gad Lubin, and Racheli Magnezi, "The Cost of Preventing Stigma by Hospitalizing Soldiers in a General Hospital Instead of a Psychiatric Hospital," *Military Medicine* 172, no. 7 (2007): 686–89.

33. Jeffrey et al., "In Service of Two Masters."

34. Jeffrey et al.

35. Tom Vanden Brook, "Army Issues Waivers to More Than 1,000 Recruits for Bipolar, Depression, Self-Mutilation," *USA Today*, April 26, 2018.

36. Tom Vanden Brook, "Army Lifts Ban on Waivers for Recruits with History of Some Mental Health Issues," *USA Today*, November 12, 2017.

37. Matthew Cox, "Army Personnel Chief: No Change in Standards for Mental Health Waivers," Military.com, November 16, 2017, https://www.military.com.

38. Human Rights Watch, *"They Want Docile": How Nursing Homes in the United States Overmedicate People with Dementia* (New York: Human Rights Watch, 2018), 36.

39. Lisa L. Dwyer, Beth Han, David A. Woodwell, and Elizabeth A. Rechtsteiner, "Polypharmacy in Nursing Home Residents in the United States: Results of the 2004 National Nursing Home Survey," *American Journal of Geriatric Pharmacotherapy* 8, no. 1 (2010): 63–72; Dorothy Gaboda, Judith Lucas, Michele Siegel, Ece Kalay, and Stephen Crystal, "No Longer Undertreated? Depression Diagnosis and Antidepressant Therapy in Elderly Long-Stay Nursing Home Residents, 1999 to 2007," *Journal of the American Geriatrics Society* 59, no. 4 (2011): 673–80.

40. Centers for Medicare and Medicaid Services, *Nursing Home Data Compendium 2012 Edition* (Washington, D.C.: U.S. Department of Health and Human Services, 2012), i–ii, http://www.cms.gov.

41. Judith Garrard, Vincent Chen, and Bryan Dowd, "The Impact of the 1987 Federal Regulations on the Use of Psychotropic Drugs in Minnesota Nursing Homes," *American Journal of Public Health* 85, no. 6 (1995): 771–76.

42. Carmel M. Hughes and Kate L. Lepane, "Administrative Initiatives for Reducing Inappropriate Prescribing of Psychotropic Drugs in Nursing Homes— How Successful Have They Been?," *Drugs & Aging* 22, no. 4 (2005): 339–51.

43. Joseph T. Hanlon, Xiaoqiang Wang, Nicholas G. Castle, Roslyn A. Stone, Steven M. Handler, Todd P. Semla, Mary Jo Pugh, Dan R. Berlowitz, and Maurice W. Dysken, "Potential Underuse, Overuse, and Inappropriate Use of Antidepressants in Older Veteran Nursing Home Residents," *Journal of the American Geriatrics Society* 59, no. 8 (2011): 1412–20.

44. Joseph T. Hanlon, Steven M. Handler, and Nicholas G. Castle, "Antidepressant Prescribing in US Nursing Homes between 1996 and 2006 and Its Relationship to Staffing Patterns and Use of Other Psychotropic Medications," *Journal of the American Medical Directors Association* 11, no. 5 (2010): 320–24.

45. Phillippe Voyer and Lori Schindel Martin, "Improving Geriatric Mental Health Nursing Care: Making a Case for Going beyond Psychotropic Medications," *International Journal of Mental Health Nursing* 12, no. 1 (2003): 11–21.

46. Julia K. Nguyen, Michelle M. Fouts, Sharon E. Kotabe, and Eunice Lo,

"Polypharmacy as a Risk Factor for Adverse Drug Reactions in Geriatric Nursing Home Residents," *American Journal of Geriatric Pharmacotherapy* 4, no. 1 (2006): 36–41.

47. Bruce K. Tamura, Christina L. Bell, Michiko Inaba, and Kamal H. Masaki, "Outcomes of Polypharmacy in Nursing Home Residents," *Clinics in Geriatric Medicine* 28, no. 2 (2012): 217–36.

48. Ann D. Bagchi, James M. Verdier, and Samuel E. Simon, "How Many Nursing Home Residents Live with a Mental Illness?," *Psychiatric Services* 60, no. 7 (2009): 958–64.

49. Victor A. Molinari, David A. Chiriboga, Laurence G. Branch, John Schinka, Lawrence Schonfeld, Lyn Kos, Whitney L. Mills, Jessica Krok, and Kathryn Hyer, "Reasons for Psychiatric Medication Prescription for New Nursing Home Residents," *Aging and Mental Health* 15, no. 7 (2011): 904–12.

50. Donald R. Hoover, Michele J. Siegel, Judith A. Lucas, Ece Kalay, Dorothy Gaboda, D. P. Devanand, and Stephen Crystal, "Depression in the First Year of Stay for Elderly Long-Term Nursing Home Residents in the USA," *International Psychogeriatrics* 22, no. 7 (2010): 1161–71.

51. Molinari et al., "Reasons for Psychiatric Medication Prescription"; Gaboda et al., "No Longer Undertreated?"; Becky A. Briesacher, M. Rhona Limcangco, Linda Simoni-Wastila, Jalpa A. Doshi, Suzi R. Levens, Dennis G. Shea, and Bruce Stuart, "The Quality of Antipsychotic Drug Prescribing in Nursing Homes," *Archives of Internal Medicine* 165, no. 11 (2005): 1280–85.

52. Molinari et al., "Reasons for Psychiatric Medication Prescription."

53. Dwyer et al., "Polypharmacy in Nursing Home Residents"; Swapna U. Karkare, Sandipan Bhattacharjee, Pravin Kamble, and Rajender Aparasu, "Prevalence and Predictors of Antidepressant Prescribing in Nursing Home Residents in the United States," *American Journal of Geriatric Pharmacotherapy* 9, no. 2 (2011): 109–19; Michele J. Siegel, Judith A. Lucas, Ayse Akincigil, Dorothy Gaboda, Donald R. Hoover, Ece Kalay, and Stephen Crystal, "Race, Education, and the Treatment of Depression in Nursing Homes," *Journal of Aging and Health* 24, no. 5 (2012): 752–78.

54. Siegel et al., "Race, Education, and the Treatment of Depression."

55. Hanlon et al., "Potential Underuse, Overuse, and Inappropriate Use of Antidepressants."

56. Pravin Kamble, Hua Chen, Jeff Sherer, and Rajender R. Aparasu, "Antipsychotic Drug Use among Elderly Nursing Home Residents in the United States," *American Journal of Geriatric Pharmacotherapy* 6, no. 4 (2008): 187–97.

57. Briesacher et al., "The Quality of Antipsychotic Drug Prescribing."

58. "Johnson & Johnson to Pay More Than $2.2. Billion to Resolve Criminal and Civil Investigations," U.S. Department of Justice, press release, November 4, 2013, http://www.justice.gov/opa/pr.

59. U.S. Department of Health and Human Services, Administration for Children and Families, Administration on Children, Youth and Families, Children's Bureau, *The AFCARS Report*, no. 20 (June 2013), https://www.acf.hhs.gov.

60. *Prescription Psychotropic Drug Use among Children in Foster Care.*

61. Curtis J. McMillen, Lionel D. Scott, Bonnie T. Zima, Marcia T. Ollie,

Michelle R. Munson, and Edward Spitznagel, "Use of Mental Health Services among Older Youths in Foster Care," *Psychiatric Services* 55, no. 7 (2004): 811–17.

62. Alfiee M. Breland-Noble, Eric B. Elbogen, Elizabeth M. Z. Farmer, Melanie S. Dubs, H. Ryan Wagner, and Barbara J. Burns, "Use of Psychotropic Medications by Youths in Therapeutic Foster Care and Group Homes," *Psychiatric Services* 55, no. 6 (2004): 706–8; Susan dosReis, Julie Magno Zito, Daniel J. Safer, and Karen L. Soeken, "Mental Health Services for Youths in Foster Care and Disabled Youths," *American Journal of Public Health* 91, no. 7 (2001): 1094–99; Michael K. Handwerk, Gail L. Smith, Ronald W. Thompson, Douglas F. Spellman, and Daniel L. Daly, "Psychotropic Medication Utilization at a Group-Home Residential Facility for Children and Adolescents," *Journal of Child and Adolescent Psychopharmacology* 18, no. 5 (2008): 517–25; Laurel K. Leslie, Ramesh Raghavan, Maia Hurley, Jinjin Zhang, John Landsverk, and Gregory Aarons, "Investigating Geographic Variation in Use of Psychotropic Medications among Youth in Child Welfare," *Child Abuse & Neglect* 35, no. 5 (2011): 333–42; David Rubin, Meredith Matone, Yuan-Shung Huang, Susan dosReis, Chris Feudtner, and Russell Localio, "Interstate Variation in Trends of Psychotropic Medication Use among Medicaid-Enrolled Children in Foster Care," *Children and Youth Services Review* 34, no. 8 (2012): 1492–99.

63. Andrés Martin, Thomas Van Hoof, Dorothy Stubbe, Tierney Sherwin, and Lawrence Scahill, "Multiple Psychotropic Pharmacotherapy among Child and Adolescent Enrollees in Connecticut Medicaid Managed Care," *Psychiatric Services* 54, no. 1 (2003): 72–77; Julie M. Zito, Daniel J. Safer, Devadatta Sai, James F. Gardner, Diane Thomas, Phyllis Coombes, Melissa Dubowski, and Maria Mendez-Lewis, "Psychotropic Medication Patterns among Youth in Foster Care," *Pediatrics* 121, no. 1 (2008): e157–63.

64. Rubin et al., "Interstate Variation in Trends of Psychotropic Medication Use."

65. Donald G. Ferguson, David C. Glesener, and Michael Raschick, "Psychotropic Drug Use with European American and American Indian Children in Foster Care," *Journal of Child and Adolescent Psychopharmacology* 16, no. 4 (2006): 474–81; Laurel K. Leslie, Ramesh Raghavan, Jinjin Zhang, and Gregory A. Aarons, "Rates of Psychotropic Medication Use over Time among Youth in Child Welfare/Child Protective Services," *Journal of Child and Adolescent Psychopharmacology* 20, no. 2 (2010): 135–43; Ramesh Raghavan and J. Curtis McMillen, "Use of Multiple Psychotropic Medications among Adolescents Aging Out of Foster Care," *Psychiatric Services* 59, no. 9 (2008): 1052–55.

66. DosReis et al., "Mental Health Services for Youths."

67. Ramesh Raghavan, Bonnie T. Zima, Ronald Max Andersen, Arleen A. Leibowitz, Mark A. Schuster, and John Landsverk, "Psychotropic Medication Use in a National Probability Sample of Children in the Child Welfare System," *Journal of Child and Adolescent Psychopharmacology* 15, no. 1 (2005): 97–106.

68. Breland-Noble et al., "Use of Psychotropic Medications by Youths."

69. Raghavan and McMillen, "Use of Multiple Psychotropic Medications."

70. Matthew M. Cummings, "Sedating Forgotten Children: How Unnecessary Psychotropic Medication Endangers Foster Children's Rights and Heath," *Boston College Journal of Law & Social Justice* 32, no. 2 (2012): 357–89.

71. Bonnie T. Zima, Regina Bussing, Gia M. Crecelius, Aaron Kaufman, and Thomas R. Belin, "Psychotropic Medication Use among Children in Foster Care: Relationship to Severe Psychiatric Disorders," *American Journal of Public Health* 89, no. 11 (1999): 1732–35.

72. Curtis J. McMillen, Nicole Fedoravicius, Jill Rowe, Bonnie T. Zima, and Norma Ware, "A Crisis of Credibility: Professionals' Concerns about the Psychiatric Care Provided to Clients of the Child Welfare System," *Administration and Policy in Mental Health and Mental Health Services Research* 34, no. 3 (2007): 203–12.

73. Julie Magno Zito, Daniel J. Safer, James F. Gardner, Laurence Magder, Karen Soeken, Myde Boles, Frances Lynch, and Mark A. Riddle, "Psychotropic Practice Patterns for Youth: A 10-Year Perspective," *Archives of Pediatrics and Adolescent Medicine* 157, no. 1 (2003): 17–25.

74. Ramesh Raghavan, Derek S. Brown, Hope Thompson, Susan L. Ettner, Lisa M. Clements, and Whitney Key, "Medicaid Expenditures on Psychotropic Medications for Children in the Child Welfare System," *Journal of Child and Adolescent Psychopharmacology* 22, no. 3 (2012): 182–89.

75. Michael W. Naylor, Christine V. Davidson, D. Jean Ortega-Piron, Arin Bass, Alice Gutierrez, and Angela Hall, "Psychotropic Medication Management for Youth in State Care: Consent, Oversight, and Policy Considerations," *Child Welfare* 86, no. 5 (2007): 175–92; Angela Olivia Burton, "'They Use It Like Candy': How the Prescription of Psychotropic Drugs to State-Involved Children Violates International Law," *Brooklyn Journal of International Law* 35, no. 2 (2010): 453–513; Rachel A. Camp, "A Mistreated Epidemic: State and Federal Failure to Adequately Regulate Psychotropic Medications Prescribed to Children in Foster Care," *Temple Law Review* 83 (2010): 369–404; Michelle L. Mello, "Psychotropic Medication and Foster Care Children: A Prescription for State Oversight," *Southern California Law Review* 85 (2011): 395–428.

76. Jeffrey Longhofer, Jerry Floersch, and Nate Okpych, "Foster Youth and Psychotropic Treatment: Where Next?," *Children and Youth Services Review* 33, no. 2 (2011): 395–404.

77. John S. Lyons and Laura Rogers, "The U.S. Child Welfare System: A De Facto Public Behavioral Health Care System," *Journal of the American Academy of Child & Adolescent Psychiatry* 43, no. 8 (2004): 971–73.

78. Dorothy Roberts, "Prison, Foster Care, and the Systematic Punishment of Black Mothers," *UCLA Law Review* 59 (2012): 1474–1500; Matthew Bramlett and Laura Radel, *Children in Non-parental Care: Findings from the 2011–2012 National Survey of Children's Health* (Washington, D.C.: U.S. Department of Health and Human Services, 2014).

79. Margaret E. Noonan and Christopher J. Mumola, *Veterans in State and Federal Prison, 2004*, BJS Special Report, NCJ 217199 (Washington, D.C.: U.S. Department of Justice, Bureau of Justice Statistics, 2007); Jack Tsai, Robert A. Rosenheck, Wesley J. Kasprow, and James F. McGuire, "Risk of Incarceration and Other Characteristics of Iraq and Afghanistan Era Veterans in State and Federal Prisons," *Psychiatric Services* 64, no. 1 (2013): 36–43; Melissa Jonson-Reid and Richard P. Barth, "From Placement to Prison: The Path to Adolescent

Incarceration from Child Welfare Supervised Foster or Group Care," *Children and Youth Services Review* 22, no. 7 (2000): 493–516; Elizabeth Johnson and Jane Waldfogel, "Parental Incarceration: Recent Trends and Implications for Child Welfare," *Social Service Review* 76, no. 3 (2002): 460–79; Joseph Doyle, "Child Protection and Adult Crime: Investigator Assignment to Estimate Causal Effects of Foster Care," *Journal of Political Economy* 116, no. 4 (2008): 746–70.

80. John Talbott, "A Special Population the Elderly Deinstitutionalized Chronically Mentally Ill Patient," *Psychiatric Quarterly* 55, nos. 2–3 (1983): 90–105; Darlene O'Connor, Faith Little, and Richard McManus, "Elders with Serious Mental Illness: Lost Opportunities and New Policy Options," *Journal of Aging and Social Policy* 21, no. 2 (2009): 144–58; David Mechanic and Donna D. McAlpine, "Use of Nursing Homes in the Care of Persons with Severe Mental Illness: 1985 to 1995," *Psychiatric Services* 51, no. 3 (2000): 354–58; Catherine Anne Fullerton, Thomas G. McGuire, Zhanlian Feng, Vincent Mor, and David C. Grabowski, "Trends in Mental Health Admissions to Nursing Homes, 1999–2005," *Psychiatric Services* 60, no. 7 (2009): 965–71.

81. Torrey et al., *More Mentally Ill Persons Are in Jails.*

82. Howard H. Goldman and Joseph P. Morrissey, "The Alchemy of Mental Health Policy: Homelessness and the Fourth Cycle of Reform," *American Journal of Public Health* 75, no. 7 (1985): 727–31; David Folsom, William Hawthorne, Laurie Lindamer, Todd Gilmer, Anne Bailey, Shahrokh Golshan, Piedad Garcia, Jürgen Unützer, Richard Hough, and Dilip V. Jeste, "Prevalence and Risk Factors for Homelessness and Utilization of Mental Health Services among 10,340 Patients with Serious Mental Illness in a Large Public Mental Health System," *American Journal of Psychiatry* 162, no. 2 (2005): 370–76.

83. Gu et al., *Prescription Drug Use Continues to Increase*; Pratt et al., *Antidepressant Use in Persons Aged 12 and Over.*

5. THERE ARE DARK DAYS AHEAD

1. Norman Carlson, testimony in *Behavior Modification Programs, Federal Bureau of Prisons, Hearing before the Subcommittee on Courts, Civil Liberties, and the Administration of Justice of the Committee on the Judiciary*, 93rd Cong., 2nd Sess. (February 27, 1974), 4.

2. Carlson, 9, quoting Harvey Wheeler, ed., *Beyond the Punitive Society: Operant Conditioning—Social and Political Aspects* (San Francisco: W. H. Freeman, 1973).

3. Peter Schrag, "Ultimate Weapons," in *Mind Control* (New York: Pantheon Books, 1978), 148–86; Andrew Scull, "Psychiatry and Social Control in the Nineteenth and Twentieth Centuries," in *The Insanity of Place/The Place of Insanity: Essays on the History of Psychiatry* (New York: Routledge, 2006), 107–28; Robert Whitaker, "Too Much Intelligence," in *Mad in America: Bad Science, Bad Medicine, and the Enduring Mistreatment of the Mentally Ill* (Cambridge: Perseus, 2002), 73–106.

4. Memorandum in Support of Motion to Enforce Class Action Lawsuit, Flores v. Sessions, Case 2:85-cv-04544-DMG-AGR, Document 409-1, filed April 16, 2018, https://www.clearinghouse.net.

5. Dana Priest and Amy Goldstein, "Suicides Point to Gaps in Treatment: Errors in Psychiatric Diagnoses and Drugs Plague Strained Immigration System," *Washington Post*, May 13, 2008, http://www.washingtonpost.com.

6. Laura Odwazny to Jocelyn Mendelsohn, U.S. Department of Health and Human Services internal memorandum, "Use of Chemical Restraints on Noncompliant Deportees," November 9, 2000.

7. Anthony S. Tangeman, director, Office of Detention and Removal, U.S. Immigration and Customs Enforcement, to ICE regional directors and assistant regional directors, U.S. Immigration and Customs Enforcement internal memorandum, "Enforcement Standard Pertaining to the Removal of Aliens under Medical Escort," May 15, 2003.

8. Amy Goldstein and Dana Priest, "Some Detainees Are Drugged for Deportation: Immigrants Sedated without Medical Reason," *Washington Post*, May 14, 2008, http://www.washingtonpost.com.

9. Thelma Gutierrez, "Lawsuit: ICE Drugging Detainees Set for Deportation," CNN, October 12, 2007, http://www.cnn.com.

10. DIHS Aviation Medicine, In-Transit Progress Notes and Medical Summary for Yousif Nageib, January 11, 2007.

11. "Information for Healthcare Professionals: Haloperidol (marketed as Haldol, Haldol Decanoate, and Haldol Lactate)," U.S. Food and Drug Administration, September 2007, http://psychrights.org.

12. Nina Bernstein, "Officials Hid Truth of Immigrant Deaths in Jail," *New York Times*, January 9, 2010.

13. Anna Gorman and Greg Kirkorian, "U.S. Officials Allegedly Drugged 2 Deportees," *Los Angles Times*, May 9, 2007, https://www.latimes.com; Paloma Esquivel, "Detainees Alleging Sedation Settle Suit," *Los Angeles Times*, January 30, 2008, https://www.latimes.com.

14. Deb Riechmann, "CIA Considered Using 'Truth Serum' on Post-9/11 Detainees," *Miami Herald*, November 18, 2018, https://www.miamiherald.com.

15. Dror Ladin, "Secret CIA Document Shows Plan to Test Drugs on Prisoners," Speak Freely (blog), American Civil Liberties Union, November 13, 2018, https://www.aclu.org.

16. Jason Leopold, "Widespread Breakdown of Safeguards at Gitmo: Military Inquiry Finds Systemic Failure Contributed to Guantanamo Prisoner's Tragic End," Al Jazeera, July 3, 2013, https://www.aljazeera.com.

17. Natalie O'Brien, "Witnesses Back Hicks on Chemical Torture," *Sydney Morning Herald*, September 16, 2012, https://www.smh.com.au.

18. Linda M. Keller, "Is Truth Serum Torture?," *American University International Law Review* 20, no. 3 (2004): 521–612.

19. Matt Apuzzo and Adam Goldman, "CIA Flight Carried Secret from Gitmo," Associated Press, August 7, 2010.

20. Peter Finn, "Defense Lawyers Get Access to Secret Guantanamo Camp," *Washington Post*, October 28, 2008; Liam Stack, "Is Waterboarding Effective? CIA Did It 266 Times on Two Prisoners," *Christian Science Monitor*, April 20, 2009.

21. Quoted in Finn, "Defense Lawyers Get Access."

22. Rasul v. Bush, 542 U.S. 466 (2004).

23. Joby Warrick, "Detainees Allege Being Drugged, Questioned," *Washington Post,* April 22, 2008. On Biden, Levin, and Hagel's call for an investigation, see Paul Kiel, "Senators Call for Investigation of Alleged Drugging of Detainees," Talking Points Memo, May 8, 2008, https://talkingpointsmemo.com.

24. Jason Leopold, "The CIA Did Not Drug Detainees before Interrogation, Says the CIA," Vice News, May 11, 2015, https://news.vice.com.

25. Gary Taylor, *Castration: An Abbreviated History of Western Manhood* (New York: Routledge, 2000).

26. Buck v. Bell, 274 U.S. 200 (1927).

27. Robert M. Foote, "Diethylstilbestrol in the Management of Psychopathological States in Males: Preliminary Report," *Journal of Nervous and Mental Disease* 99, no. 6 (1944): 928–35.

28. John Bradford, "The Hormonal Treatment of Sexual Offenders," *Journal of the American Academy of Psychiatry and the Law* 11, no. 2 (1983): 159–69; John Money, "Use of an Androgen-Depleting Hormone in the Treatment of Male Sex Offenders," *Journal of Sex Research* 6, no. 3 (1970): 165–72.

29. Gregory Lehne and John Money, "The First Case of Paraphilia Treated with Depo-Provera: 40-Year Outcome," *Journal of Sex Education and Therapy* 25, no. 4 (2000): 213–20.

30. Alessandro Tagliamonte, Paola Tagliamonte, Gian L. Gessa, and Bernard B. Brodie, "Compulsive Sexual Activity Induced by p-Chlorophenylalanine in Normal and Pinealectomized Male Rats," *Science* 166, no. 3911 (December 12, 1969): 1433–35.

31. Boris B. Gorzalka, Scott D. Mendelson, and Neil V. Watson, "Serotonin Receptor Subtypes and Sexual Behavior," *Annals of the New York Academy of Sciences* 600, no. 1 (1990): 435–44; James G. Pfaus and Barry J. Everitt, "The Psychopharmacology of Sexual Behavior," in *Psychopharmacology: The Fourth Generation of Progress,* ed. Floyd E. Bloom and David J. Kupfer (New York: Raven Press, 1995), 743–58. On the monoamine hypothesis, see Martin P. Kafka, "The Monoamine Hypothesis for the Pathophysiology of Paraphilic Disorders: An Update," *Annals of the New York Academy of Sciences* 989, no. 1 (2003): 86–94; Martin P. Kafka, "A Monoamine Hypothesis for the Pathophysiology of Paraphilic Disorders," *Archives of Sexual Behavior* 26, no. 4 (1997): 343–58.

32. The monoamine hypothesis is now incorporated in R. Karl Hanson and Kelly Morton-Bourgon, *Predictors of Sexual Recidivism: An Updated Meta-Analysis* (Ottawa: Public Works and Government Services Canada, 2004). This frequently cited publication has informed a range of sex offender management assessments and treatment regimes.

33. "Pharmacological Interventions with Adult Male Sexual Offenders," Association for the Treatment of Sexual Abusers, August 30, 2012, http://www.atsa.com.

34. Bradley Booth, "How to Select Pharmacologic Treatments to Manage Recidivism Risk in Sex Offenders," *Current Psychiatry* 8, no. 10 (2009): 60–67.

35. Stacy Anderson Light and Suzanne Holroyd, "The Use of Medroxyprogesterone Acetate for the Treatment of Sexually Inappropriate Behaviour in

Patients with Dementia," *Journal of Psychiatry and Neuroscience* 31, no. 2 (2006): 132–34.

36. Robert J. McGrath, Georgia F. Cumming, Brenda L. Burchard, Stephen Zeoli, and Lawrence Ellerby, *Current Practices and Emerging Trends in Sexual Abuser Management: The Safer Society 2009 North American Survey* (Brandon, Vt.: Safer Society Press, 2010), 75.

37. Booth, "How to Select Pharmacologic Treatments," 61.

38. Yaser Adi, D. Ashcroft, Kevin Browne, Anthony Beech, A. Fry-Smith, and Christopher Hyde, "Clinical Effectiveness and Cost-Consequences of Selective Serotonin Reuptake Inhibitors in the Treatment of Sex Offenders," *Health Technology Assessment* 6, no. 28 (2002): 1–66.

39. Martin Kafka, cited in Lauren Slater, "How Do You Cure a Sex Addict," *New York Times Magazine*, November 19, 2000, 96–102.

40. John M. W. Bradford, "The Neurobiology, Neuropharmacology, and Pharmacological Treatment of the Paraphilias and Compulsive Sexual Behaviour," *Canadian Journal of Psychiatry* 46, no. 1 (2001): 26–34.

41. Daniel Turner, Julius Petermann, Karen Harrison, Richard Krueger, and Peer Briken, "Pharmacological Treatment of Patients with Paraphilic Disorders and Risk of Sexual Offending: An International Perspective," *World Journal of Biological Psychiatry* (2017): 1–10.

42. Healy et al., "Antidepressants and Violence"; Moore et al., "Prescription Drugs Associated with Reports of Violence"; Breggin, *Medication Madness*.

43. "Encounter Report" faxed from Ashley Zelaya of the Altamonte Family Practice to Investigator Sirino of the Sanford Police Department, dated March 9, 2012, https://blackbutterfly7.files.wordpress.com/2013/09/george-zimmermans -medical-record.pdf.

44. Rene Stutzman, "George Zimmerman's Father: My Son Is Not Racist, Did Not Confront Trayvon Martin," *Orlando Sentinel*, March 15, 2012. Zimmerman's racial and ethnic identity are contested. While he has become widely identified as white, to be essentialist about it, he is non-Hispanic white and Peruvian, as reported by his father, according to this *Orlando Sentinel* article. See also the discussion of Zimmerman's race and ethnicity in Julianne King, "The Curious Case of George Zimmerman's Race," Colorlines, July 22, 2013, https://www .colorlines.com.

45. Richard Hammersley and Stephanie Pearl, "Temazepam Misuse, Violence and Disorder," *Addiction Research* 5, no. 3 (1997): 213–22.

46. Judith Aldridge, "Decline but No Fall? New Millennium Trends in Young People's Use of Illegal and Illicit Drugs in Britain," *Health Education* 108, no. 3 (2008): 189–206.

47. Stephanie Saul, "F.D.A. Issues Warning on Sleeping Pills," *New York Times*, March 15, 2007.

48. "Dextroamphetamine and Amphetamine," MedlinePlus, last revised September 15, 2017, https://medlineplus.gov.

49. Moore et al., "Prescription Drugs Associated with Reports of Violence."

50. "Librax," WebMD, https://www.webmd.com.

51. "Chlordiazepoxide," MedlinePlus, last revised April 15, 2017, https:// medlineplus.gov.

52. "Chlordiazepoxide/clidinium drug interactions," Drugs.com, https://www.drugs.com.

53. Serge Kovaleski, "Trayvon Martin Case Shadowed by Series of Police Missteps," *New York Times*, May 12, 2012.

54. Florida Department of Law Enforcement Agency Reports 20125001136 (March 21, 2012) and 2012051890 (March 26, 2012), Exhibit JR-2.

55. Tracy Connor and Daniel Arkin, "Police Called to Incident between George Zimmerman, Wife," September 9, 2013, https://www.nbcnews.com.

56. Salamishah Tillet, "Domestic Violence and George Zimmerman's Defense," Police and Law Enforcement (blog), *The Nation*, July 15, 2013, http://www.thenation.com; Jonathan Capeheart, "George Zimmerman's Relevant Past," PostPartisan (blog), *Washington Post*, May 28, 2013, http://www.washingtonpost.com.

57. Richard Luscombe, "George Zimmerman Domestic Violence Charges Dropped," *The Guardian*, December 11, 2013, http://www.theguardian.com.

58. Danielle Canada, "George Zimmerman, Son of a Retired Judge, Has 3 Closed Arrests," Rollingout.com, March 27, 2012, http://rollingout.com.

59. Barbara Liston, "George Zimmerman's Medical Records Targeted on Eve of Hearing," *Chicago Tribune*, October 18, 2012, https://www.chicagotribune.com.

60. According to the National Council of State Legislatures, eight U.S. states do not currently prohibit the sale of firearms to persons who have been deemed mentally incompetent or who have been institutionalized: North Carolina, Idaho, Montana, New Hampshire, Vermont, Tennessee, Alabama, and Arkansas.

61. Urara Hiroeh, Louis Appleby, Preben Bo Mortensen, and Graham Dunn, "Death by Homicide, Suicide, and Other Unnatural Causes in People with Mental Illness: A Population-Based Study," *The Lancet*, 358, no. 9299 (December 2001): 2110–12; Linda A. Teplin, Gary M. McClelland, Karen M. Abram, and Dana A. Weiner, "Crime Victimization in Adults with Severe Mental Illness: Comparison with the National Crime Victimization Survey," *Archives of General Psychiatry* 62, no. 8 (2005): 911–21.

62. 18 U.S.C. 922(d).

63. "Health Insurance Portability and Accountability Act (HIPAA) Privacy Rule and the National Instant Criminal Background Check System (NICS)," rule by the Department of Health and Human Services, January 6, 2016, effective February 5, 2016, https://www.federalregister.gov.

64. "Possession of Firearms by People with Mental Illness," National Council of State Legislatures, January 5, 2018, http://www.ncsl.org.

65. Andy Mannix, "At Urging of Minneapolis Police, Hennepin EMS Workers Subdued Dozens with a Powerful Sedative," *Star Tribune* (Minneapolis), June 15, 2018.

CONCLUSION

1. "The Science of Drug Use and Addiction: The Basics," National Institute on Drug Abuse, updated July 2018, https://www.drugabuse.gov; American Psychiatric Association, *Diagnostic and Statistical Manual of Mental Disorders*, 5th ed. (Arlington, Va.: American Psychiatric Association, 2013).

2. Citizens United v. Federal Election Commission, 558 U.S. 310 (2010).

3. Benjamin Rush, *Medical Inquiries and Observations upon the Diseases of the Mind* (Philadelphia: Grigg and Elliot, 1812), 181.

4. Michel Foucault, *Psychiatric Power: Lectures at the Collège de France, 1973–1974,* ed. Jacques Lagrange, trans. Graham Burchell (New York: Palgrave Macmillan, 2006), 184–95. The five tokens of knowledge that Foucault describes are as follows: (1) the doctor must know more about the patient than the patient himself knows; (2) the doctor must question the patient incessantly and force him to answer; (3) the doctor and the institution must keep a documentary record, a file, on the patient that accounts for every interaction between doctor and patient; (4) the doctor must use medication and direction together to obscure the relationship between the two; and (5) the doctor must use the questioning of the patient to teach medical students.

5. Foucault, 185.

6. Foucault, 189.

7. Foucault, 189.

8. Nick Crossley, "R. D. Laing and the British Anti-psychiatry Movement: A Socio-historical Analysis," *Social Science & Medicine* 47, no. 7 (1998): 877–89; Marcelo Berlim, Marcelo Fleck, and Edward Shorter, "Notes on Antipsychiatry," *European Archives of Psychiatry and Clinical Neuroscience* 253, no. 2 (2003): 61–67; Peter Sedgwick, *Psychopolitics* (New York: Harper & Row, 1982); Thomas Szasz, *Psychiatry: The Science of Lies* (Syracuse, N.Y.: Syracuse University Press, 2008); Foucault, *Psychiatric Power*; Franco Basaglia, *Psychiatry Inside Out: Selected Writings of Franco Basaglia,* ed. Nancy Scheper-Hughes and Anne M. Lovell, trans. Teresa Shtob (New York: Columbia University Press, 1987).

9. "About Our Agency," Federal Bureau of Prisons, https://www.bop.gov.

10. Alexander, *The New Jim Crow.*

11. For further development of this view of carceral technologies by an interdisciplinary group of scholars, see Ruha Benjamin, ed., *Captivating Technology: Race, Carceral Technoscience, and Liberatory Imagination in Everyday Life* (Durham, N.C.: Duke University Press, 2019).

12. Langdon Winner, "Do Artifacts Have Politics?," *Daedalus* 109, no. 1 (1980): 134.

13. Fannie Lou Hamer, interview by George Foster in "The Heritage of Slavery," episode of the documentary television series *Of Black America* (New York: Phoenix/BFA Films & Video, 1968).

INDEX

ANTHONY RYAN HATCH is associate professor in the Science in Society Program at Wesleyan University. He is the author of *Blood Sugar: Racial Pharmacology and Food Justice in Black America* (Minnesota, 2016).